MANAGEMENT FOR DOCTORS

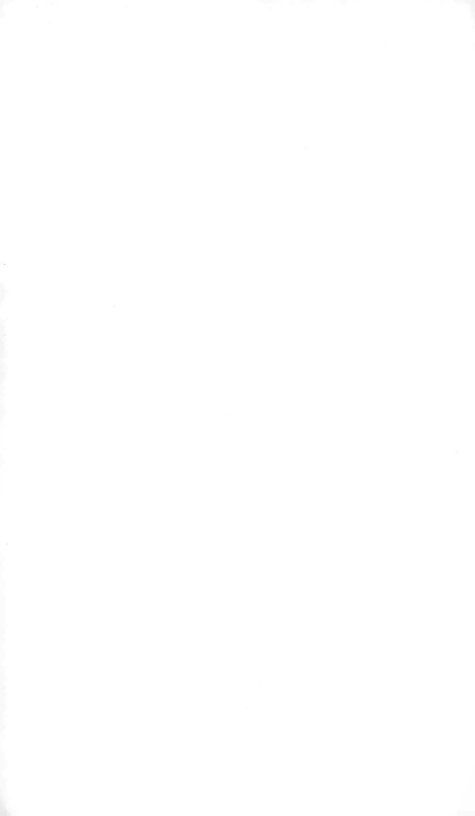

MANAGEMENT FOR DOCTORS

Edited by Jenny Simpson, *chief executive,*
British Association of Medical Managers
and Richard Smith, *editor, British Medical Journal*

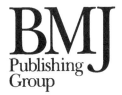

First published in 1995
by the BMJ Publishing Group, BMA House, Tavistock Square,
London WC1H 9JR

British Library Cataloguing in Publication Data

A catalogue record for this book is available
from the British Library

ISBN 0-7279-0858–8

Typeset in Great Britain by Apek Typesetters Ltd., Nailsea, Bristol
Printed and bound in Great Britain by Latimer Trend & Company Ltd, Plymouth, Devon

Contents

Introduction

Most doctors regard management as boring. Why should anybody want to fret about budgets, staff, and strategy when they could be replacing heart valves, tending to the dying, or researching into the molecular pathology of disease? Management is for doctors who are too old and burnt out for anything better.

This used to be my view. As a young assistant editor, I looked at my seniors and pitied them. Where was the joy in management? But then I spent a year at the Stanford Business School in California and changed my view completely. I now see management as enormously creative. It may be difficult, demanding, complex, and exhausting – and bring you far fewer plaudits than treating patients or writing editorials – but it offers you an opportunity to achieve with others far more than you could ever hope to achieve on your own. No matter how clever you are you cannot hope to introduce a new service into a hospital, raise the quality of asthma care within a health centre, or reduce deaths from heart disease in a region without understanding something of the techniques of management.

This book will not make you a manager, but it will provide you with some insights if you know nothing of management and help you organise your thinking if you know a little; it should also stimulate you, perhaps through disagreement, even if you know a lot. You will also be helped to understand something of the challenges that managers face and so perhaps understand their difficulties. Because one of the gravest threats to the health service in Britain and other countries is the inability of doctors and managers to work together. A moment's thought will show that

1

the long term future of the health service depends on doctors and managers cooperating.

Sir Maurice Shock, former rector of Lincoln College, Oxford, when invited to open a summit meeting of British doctors' leaders in November 1994, said: "You must participate directly in the management of the health service. There have been far too few doctors prepared to move into management. Those who do it have got to be good doctors. It is no good having those who have dropped out because their medicine was not up to the mark. You have also got to put your backs into ensuring that managers – whether doctors or not – are properly trained."

Similarities between managers and doctors

Although we hear so much about the differences between doctors and managers in the health service, I believe that they are more similar than dissimilar. For a start, both professions expect considerable commitment. Doctors are prone to the error of thinking that they are the only people who work hard, but many managers are to be found working late into the night and at weekends. Indeed, both groups probably put too much emphasis on hard work – to the point of damaging themselves and their families.

I also believe that management has, like medicine, high ethical values. Both professions have their quacks, rogues, and malcontents, but most business schools include a substantial course on ethics. Many graduates from business school work in developing countries or in public sector management. Those high quality managers who work in the NHS are working for substantially less than they would earn in the private sector, and unlike some doctors they cannot top up their NHS salaries with a large private income. Managers respond to financial rewards, but so do doctors: the response to item of service payments has shown this time and time again. Doctors mustn't make the mistake of thinking that they are the only profession with high ethical standards.

Doctors have a long, intensive training – but so do many managers. It is harder to get into the business school at Stanford than into the medical school, and the two year graduate master of business administration course demands 80 hours' study a week.

It is, however, one of the failings of management in Britain and in the NHS that few managers have formal, high quality training.

Managers are also like doctors in undertaking widely different jobs. Medicine has a core set of skills and so does management, but just as neurosurgeons need different skills than public health doctors so finance directors are different from human resource managers. Simon Weill said that all sentences that begin with "we" are lies, and sentences that begin "doctors" or "managers" must be treated cautiously.

Successful doctors, just like successful managers, tend to be people of action. Both professions need time to reflect, but action predominates. Communication is also important in both professions, no matter whether you are telling a woman that she is dying or a man that he is fired. And both professions use too much jargon and are inclined to speak and write pompously and opaquely. Both are regularly criticised for their poor communication.

Both medicine and management tend to be dominated by middle aged men, and it is hard for women to advance in both professions. Travel and international activity are common among doctors and managers, and both professions have their fair share of risk takers.

The senior members of both professions are also very alike in their lifestyles, tending to vote conservative, wear suits and ties, enjoy sport and middlebrow culture, take foreign holidays, send their children to private schools, and drink too much. Doctors and managers who row in the local newspapers may well belong to the same Masonic lodge.

What doctors can teach managers

Medicine has a stronger intellectual base than management, and the best medicine is rooted in science – despite the increasing recognition of the lack of rigorous evidence of effectiveness in medicine. Economics and finance are strong intellectual disciplines that lie at the base of management, but marketing and strategic management are fledgling academic disciplines. Many doctors are frustrated by the lack of research evidence to support much of what the management gurus say – but so are many managers. Management needs to strengthen its research base, and doctors may be able to help. Doctors can also help managers by teaching them more about the parts of medicine that will be useful to them – for instance, methods for determining the effectiveness of new treatments or diagnostic methods.

Medicine is an ancient profession, while management is a young one. But it isn't so long since doctors were barbers and apothecaries, and the age of organisations within medicine – the General Medical Council and the royal colleges, for instance, in Britain – may bring problems as well as benefits. Management might, however, benefit from having more and better systems of self regulation. Doctors could help.

One of the great strengths of medicine is that its most senior members deal regularly with individuals – patients. Senior managers are often very remote from the customer, despite paying lip service to his or her importance. Managers could learn from doctors about the importance of staying in touch with customers and the "front line" of the business.

Doctors are much more individualistic than managers and feel happiest in flat structures, which modern management is now encouraging. Doctors perhaps overvalue autonomy, but managers may be too quick to put the organisation first.

A final lesson that doctors might teach managers – and I would say this, wouldn't I? – is about the importance of a written culture. Medical journals might contain a lot of rubbish and some young doctors might be forced to publish for career advancement when they have nothing interesting to say, but a written culture allows high quality debate and intellectual development that is not easily matched by a predominantly oral culture, which is what managers have.

What managers can teach doctors

Managers understand strategic thinking in a way that doctors do not. Doctors tend to be driven by science and suffering to act tactically rather than strategically. Similarly doctors tend to be poor leaders and are suspicious of those who purport to be leaders. But leaders can make things happen by setting a clear vision and motivating people to want to achieve that objective. Doctors need to examine their attitudes to leadership, and managers could help them.

Doctors are more awkward in teams and organisations than managers, which is a problem because in this increasingly complex world most important tasks – no matter whether it's transplanting livers or marketing contraceptives to young people – depend on teamwork. Doctors say that they believe in teams but are inclined to see other members of the team as people who help them rather than themselves as equal members of the team.

Most doctors have a very limited understanding of economics, accountancy, finance, and budgets, and what's worse they are often proud of their ignorance. But economic and financial pressures drive the modern world, and doctors are handicapped by this ignorance. Not all doctors need a profound knowledge of these sometimes arcane matters, but I believe that any educated person should in addition to knowing something of language, mathematics, science, history, and geography know something about economics.

Managers also have something to teach doctors about negotiation, conflict resolution, organisational psychology, and selling and marketing. Many doctors may believe that these disciplines have nothing useful to offer them, but wouldn't you like to be able, for instance, to market a healthy lifestyle more effectively to your patients?

What makes a good manager?

Defining what characterises a good doctor is hard, and it's just as difficult to define a good manager. Nevertheless, attempts have been made to identify the qualities of a good manager; what follows is the result of a study of managers at Maxwell House in the United States. Jim was identified by other managers in the company as the best manager, and these are his characteristics. (I have to observe that a study conducted in 1994 would probably identify a woman as the best manager, but this study was done a dozen years ago.)

Jim's most important asset in the eyes of his fellow managers was that he was a doer and a solver of problems. He got on and did things, following the philosophy that "it's much easier to beg forgiveness than to ask permission." He was a self confident optimist but far from being a braggart.

He could describe in detail his strategy for "being number

one," and he had a detailed knowledge of what competitors were doing. He was fiercely loyal to the company and loved nothing better than to "clobber" the opposition. Although a disciplinarian who defined clearly for his staff their range of freedom, he listened to the advice of those below him; and he would never let preconceptions get in the way of understanding what his staff were telling him. He was a great motivator of people, identifying what people wanted from their jobs, but he was also good at setting priorities.

A great salesman, he ignored irrelevant paperwork but dealt efficiently with the administrative tasks that had to be done. He fitted into his environment but what he didn't like he changed. Finally, he lived very much for today and would recover instantly from a bruising battle that he had lost.

This example was given to me at the Stanford Business School in 1989, and as I sketch it out now I feel it is old fashioned. To some extent Jim is the outdated "heroic" manager who feels that he must be in charge of everything and take all the important decisions. Modern managers are much more likely to let the team take the important decisions and put considerable energy into ensuring the effectiveness of the team and the clarity of its objectives; but perhaps the managers of 10 years hence will be different again.

One thing that is clear to me is that all managers have their own style and must to a large extent follow that style. If managers who are effective when directing others switch to being democratic because it is more fashionable they may well fail. You must understand your own strengths and weaknesses.

The history of this book

This book is not directive. It does contain practical advice, but it aims primarily to expose doctors to the problems encountered in modern management within the NHS and to some ideas on how they might be solved. This case study method of teaching is popular in management education because it recognises that little is clearly right or wrong, that each predicament demands different actions, and that there are many different ways to be effective.

The book has had a long and difficult gestation. We had what seemed at the time the bright idea of asking a doctor who had some experience of management to team up with a business academic who could ensure that what was said was up to date and correct. We were also keen that each chapter should contain a case to which most doctors would be able to relate. In a very few cases this model worked quickly and well, but more often the doctors and academics found it difficult to work together and it proved difficult to get the tone of the cases and articles just right.

But in the end we got there, and I hope that doctors and other health workers will find that this book stimulates them to think seriously about management and to recognise that far from being dull it can be one of life's most rewarding activities.

RICHARD SMITH
Editor, *BMJ*
November 1994

1 Doctors and management—why bother?

JENNY SIMPSON

Case study

In November the chief executive of St Christopher's, Mr Vincent, announced that the oncology ward would be closed for five months from the following week, for redecoration. Medical staff were outraged: this ward provided specialist oncology care for children from all over the region, and their parents gained a good deal of support, both from each other and from the medical staff. The oncology service had been built up over many years and provided specialist training courses for nursing and other staff.

Patients were to be dispersed around the general wards and thus put at considerable risk of infection. Staff were also sure that the specialist nurses would find work in other oncology units and so the hospital would lose its oncology nursing expertise. The consultants' anger was further fuelled by the fact that, on the face of things, doctors were being encouraged to take part in management, an involvement vociferously endorsed by the general manager. The hospital had a clinical directorate structure, although very little in the way of significant decisions seemed to be discussed at the clinical directors' meetings. The atmosphere had become increasingly sour over the previous two years, and several highly respected clinicians had left for posts in the pharmaceutical industry and abroad.

The following week several consultants challenged Mr Vincent about his decision. He explained that he had taken advice from some senior key clinicians, but refused to name them. This resulted in much speculation, suspicion, and ill feeling among the consultants. The nurses were also furious and felt that they had been betrayed by trusted colleagues. The atmosphere was extremely tense, and at the end of the week Dr Roberts called a meeting of the medical staff.

At the meeting it transpired that no one had, in fact, advised Mr Vincent about the subject of the oncology ward. All the consultants agreed that the situation was unacceptable, but were somehow at a loss as to how to resolve it. They took advice from a wide range of sources, including the trust chairman, who came to the conclusion that the relationship between Mr Vincent and the clinical directors would not support the successful operation of the trust. Mr Vincent was redeployed, while Mr Parker, a pathologist with many years' experience of chairing medical staff and a number of district and regional committees, took over as chief executive.

The management process in the hospital rapidly improved, as did the consultants' morale. But things were not so comfortable for Dr Roberts. Shortly after Mr Vincent took up his new post, Dr Roberts was summoned to the chairman's office. The chairman had been very supportive of Dr Roberts's involvement, but now told him that he had been a disruptive influence in the hospital, that he was "far too articulate" in meetings, and that he should leave the hospital that afternoon.

Learning points from the case

(1) The key relationship between chief executive and clinical professionals

No matter how sophisticated the clinical professionals' technical skills or how loyal and committed of the hospital staff, unless both management and clinical professionals share a single set of values and ideals about the ultimate goals and proper functioning of the organisation, it will never flourish. The mismatch in attitude at St Christopher's between clinical staff and the chief executive had resulted in a distrustful atmosphere, which eventually permeated the entire organisation, making it an unpleasant place in which to work. In these circumstances, talented staff leave and it is difficult to attract high calibre new applicants to replace them. Managerial skill on the part of the chief executive, managerial commitment on the part of the clinical professionals, and determination to develop a trusting respectful relationship by both managers and clinicians are essential preconditions for the longterm strategic health of a hospital.

(2) Decision making should be explicit and information-based

Effective decision making in today's health care organisations is made on the basis of explicit information. Clinicians form a valuable source of information and expertise, which Mr Vincent failed to use in his decision making. They expect to be part of the explicit and information based processes. Considerable unrest ensues if this does not happen. As technology advances, the arguments of five or 10 years ago, of the information simply not being available, are no longer tenable.

(3) Decentralisation on paper must be borne out in practice and by management processes

Decentralisation of management responsibility to clinical resource centres entails a true devolution of management authority. Decentralised organisation structures can function only if those leading clinical services are sufficiently empowered and supported by central management to make significant and far reaching changes in the organisation of their own services, and to make a contribution to the management of the hospital as a whole.

Failure to devolve management authority leads to scepticism among clinical staff, who feel that they have taken on the blame for any overspending, but are powerless to do anything about it. This rapidly leads to disenchantment and distrust, and, as took place at St Christopher's, a deterioration in what may already be vulnerable relationships.

(4) The power of working as a team

Doctors are not, by culture or tradition, strong corporate team players. The nature of their profession, with ultimate named responsibility for individual patients, dictates an organisation of single players, albeit supported by their own teams of juniors. This means that many doctors gain little experience of working as equal players in teams. The exceptions are those who work across specialties—for example, in intensive care or in rehabilitation units. To work effectively in a team requires a different set of skills from those required as a single player, and not all doctors manage to acquire these skills. Sometimes, however, as at St Christopher's, the clinical staff are galvanised into adopting strong corporate behaviour by adversity, and once team behaviour is established, it can be developed further.

A group of clinicians working effectively together on management issues is far more powerful than a single voice and can often bring about major change. But such effective corporate behaviour can also be perceived as extremely threatening to the management, and can result in reactive behaviour, which can be seriously disruptive. In the case study Dr Roberts was seen by management as being responsible for loss of managerial control, and most particularly for Mr Vincent's downfall, and was duly removed.

The doctor in management — setting the scene

Hospitals have a complex organisational structure in which professional providers of the service and managers of the infrastructure cohabit, with varying degrees of harmony. Hospitals are far from straightforward to manage.

As in other service industries, the quality of the "product" of health care is determined by the expert skills and knowledge of the front line workers—the clinicians—who, by every decision they make, commit whatever resources are available. The non-clinical managers cannot directly control their activity. Thus the mechanisms for managing in a manufacturing context - where hierarchical control and decision making by those with a superior knowledge base (at the top of the organisation) is exercised over the less skilled and knowledgeable front line workers - do not apply. Tensions between professionals and managers are inevitable and can either catalyse the formation of strong and effective teams of doctors, nurses, other professionals, and managers or, as at St Christopher's, can be mishandled and destroy any possibility of working together.

Today's clinicians and managers work in an environment that has evolved since 1983, when Sir Roy Griffiths responded to the NHS Management Inquiry, "the nearer that the management process gets to the patient, the more important it becomes for doctors to be looked upon as the natural managers."[1] The decision facing the manager centres on the extent to which he or she is prepared to devolve the centralised power base of longterm decision making, budgets, resource allocation, and information to those more directly involved in patient care. By devolution,

11

however, the manager is not absolved of the final responsibility for the proper functioning of the organisation. The reason that health care provision demands an extremely high calibre of manager is that it is, indeed, difficult to devolve power, authority, and budget responsibility while at the same time retaining a leadership position.

Involvement in management for the clinician can be a time consuming, emotionally draining, and at times, nerve racking experience. Time devoted to management activities, let alone education, is inevitably in conflict with either clinical or private time, and in an unsupportive organisation may have no financial reward. Yet doctors are increasingly taking on the roles of clinical director, medical director, or other clinical and management combinations. Furthermore, these doctors, while initially perhaps being motivated by a sense of duty, are now keen to improve their management skills and enthusiastic to continue in their new roles. Indeed, some who have completed a fixed term—for example, as a clinical director—have found the experience so rewarding that they wish to continue, and in some cases make a permanent career move. Many doctors find that dealing with the wider picture, gaining the opportunity to influence the organisation as a whole and the direction it will take, provides a refreshing and stimulating challenge, particularly when set against the perspective of their clinical duties. They find that solving management problems appeals to their creative talents and is both exciting and challenging.

Doctors must decide for themselves how much time and energy they will invest in a managerial role and the learning process required to make a meaningful contribution. The role of any senior clinical practitioner has managerial components - achieving goals through motivating others, monitoring and developing the performance of juniors, making complex longterm decisions, and organising workload. There is a strong argument for education on management for all doctors at both undergraduate and postgraduate levels. However, the decision to take on an active role in hospital management should not be undertaken lightly, nor without a clear understanding not only of the demands and nature of the task but also of the considerable rewards. Doctors must also think carefully of the consequences of not being involved in management, at an individual as well as a professional level.

How have doctors and managers traditionally regarded each other?

In the past doctors may have perceived in managers a value system driven by a need to keep the district or regional headquarters happy, making decisions that were politically and financially acceptable rather than being driven by patients' needs or the quality of their care. Decisions were often perceived as being taken behind closed doors by some mysterious process and then delivered to the medical staff, with or without the veneer of a consultative process. Furthermore, the perception was commonly held that a "management mafia" existed, designed to keep the manager commited to "not rocking the boat," in position to increase the control of district (as it was then) and regional headquarters. Such views were widely held at St Christopher's.

For the manager's part, doctors in many instances have been regarded as an unruly bunch of mavericks with more power than is desirable and no sense of responsibility for the hospital as a whole. Medical staff have been perceived as extremely poor team players, interested only in their own clinical empires with very little appreciation of the world outside medicine and the environment in which the organisation exists. In many instances management have taken something of a patronising stance, ridiculing doctors' lack of awareness and management acumen.

The lack of a common dialogue between doctors and managers has led to considerable frustration in many clinicians. At St Christopher's the consultants felt that their intimate and expert knowledge of the systems and processes, the business of the hospital, was wasted as they were unable to effect any significant change within the organisation. This sort of situation is not helped by the tradition of senior doctors tending to stay in the same institution for many years, often for their total career, gaining little experience of other management cultures and limiting their understanding of the possibilities for change.

Ten years on from the Griffiths inquiry, and influenced in great measure by the more recent initiatives of *Resource Management* and *Working for Patients*, there has been a dramatic change in attitude on the parts of both doctors and managers. In many parts of the country the old relationships are barely recognisable. However, the changes are by no means uniform; there are still some hospitals in which suspicion and distrust predominate.

Medical managers — leaders or administrators?

> *All leadership is show business. All management is show business. That doesn't mean tap dancing; it means shaping values, symbolising attention — and it is the opposite of administration.*
>
> Tom Peters[2]

Management is concerned with getting things done through influencing others. It is concerned with making decisions, not only on a day to day basis, but also longterm, strategic decisions which determine the direction that the service or organisation will take. The doctor in management must learn to be a team player, but also take on a leadership role among his or her colleagues. Charles Handy defines the leader as someone who "shapes and shares a vision which gives point to the work of others."[3] The leader must describe and develop a vision of precisely why the organisation exists, to what end, for whose benefit. In the light of this definition the leader must examine every single structure, process, and approach to making decisions and all the activities that make up the hospital organisation, and if necessary redesign them to ensure that they are geared towards supporting this ideal. At St Christopher's Dr Roberts took on this role in the course of the organisational changes largely because Mr Vincent did not; there was a leadership vacuum which eventually required resolution.

> *The leader — cheerleader, enthusiast, nurturer of champions, hero finder, wanderer dramatist, coach, facilitator, builder.*
>
> *Leadership by means of passion, care, intensity, consistency, attention, drama, using implicit and explicit symbols.*
>
> Tom Peters[4]

The traditional perspectives and skills of doctors—observation, analysis, diagnosis, problem solving, and developing action plans—when applied to the broader picture of the organisation as a whole rather than to a specific patient, serve as an effective framework on which to base management and understanding of leadership. There is no mystique to management: its subject matter, approaches, and language may be readily learnt by interested doctors and translated into the health care environment. To be an effective leader requires an intimate understanding of the structures in the organisation: its anatomy (an understanding of the system); its physiology (the systems and processes); and the environment in which it exists.

Understanding the anatomy

The structure of an organisation plays a major part in determining how it works and with what effect. The structure defines who reports to whom and the levels at which decisions are made. Hospitals are complex entities in managerial terms, considerably more complex than one would be led to believe by either the status of management in health care in the United Kingdom or the emphasis placed on investment in educating or training of managers of appropriate calibre.

Hospitals are not simple, hierarchical structures, but, along with universities and other educational establishments, fall into the category of "professional bureaucracy" as defined by Mintzberg.[5] This type of structure is characterised by a central operating core of the most highly skilled and intensively trained individuals (the clinical staff providing the service for patients). The management role in this type of bureaucracy is to underpin the professional activity and to ensure that the "product," in this case the clinical process, is supported by groups of appropriate and effectively functioning staff. The non-professional manager cannot control the activities of the professional operating core and must therefore adopt a very different management style from that of an executive in a production orientated hierarchical environment.

The involvement of clinicians in the management process formalises and makes explicit the need for the professional body to make responsible and informed management decisions which will have a significant impact on the functioning of the organisation as a whole. Although the concept of decentralising the controlling role of management and the terms "supportive" and "co-ordinating," might initially be perceived as requiring a weaker, less skilled manager, this is far from the case. The professional bureaucracy demands a skilled, sensitive manager who is capable of leading from the side, drawing on the skills and leadership qualities of the medical and nursing staff and pulling the decentralised clinical teams together to form an effective, corporate whole. Had Mr Vincent been prepared to take a less autocratic stance, and behaved more as a co-ordinator, the

15

situation at St Christopher's may well have been averted, if a single decision making body had been established. This would have allowed all the clinical directors and the management executive to make any decision together concerning the running of the hospital, as advocated in *Managing Clinical Services.*[5]

Understanding the physiology

Running hospitals involves complex processes. Set against the wider political organisation of the NHS as a whole, the organisational issues become ever more complicated, posing a considerable challenge to anyone attempting to disentangle the basic processes of decision making, financial allocation, and policy making. However, an understanding of these systems and processes, of how things happen in the NHS, is essential to the clinician who wishes to make a truly effective contribution to management, and greatly increases his or her chances of influencing either the input, the process, or the output. Most importantly, the clinician needs to understand the systems by which: information flows through the organisation; decisions are made; and decision making is communicated and implemented throughout the organisation.

Peter Drucker, a leading authority on management processes for the past 50 years, has identified five areas of expertise required for effective management.[6]

In the world of trusts and clinical directorates many of the convoluted processes and multiple levels at which decisions were made within individual systems have been replaced by a more direct form of both operational and strategic decision making. This should result in more straightforward processes, with those

---

Drucker's five talents for effectiveness in management

(1) Time management

(2) Identifying the particular contribution to the organisation

(3) Identifying where and how to apply particular strengths to best effort

(4) Setting the right priorities

(5) Effective decision making

---

who are expected to implement decisions much more closely involved in the way they are made. However, not all provider units are undergoing instant and complete change. Many, as at St Christopher's, where clinical directors were in place but not making any effective contribution to the management process, exhibit both old style and new style management arrangements simultaneously, somewhat to the confusion of the clinical staff. A more detailed appreciation of the process at work at St Christopher's by the consultant staff would perhaps have resulted in a less traumatic series of events.

The environment

Not only are the structures and processes of health care management complex, but the environment, both internal and external, of health care provider units is also far from stable. It is an inescapable fact that health care in the United Kingdom, as in many other countries, is inextricably linked with political issues, and the effects of this are felt at all levels of the service. Technological advance has a widespread influence on both clinical activity and consumption of resources, and published effectiveness and outcomes information may significantly alter the course of clinical practice. At a more local level, a wide range of external environmental factors affects the way in which the organisation functions—for example, its location or the personality and disposition of key purchasers.

In terms of internal environments, there may well be power struggles—between groups of clinicians or between clinicians and management—which can undermine the organisation's operations. An understanding of all the dimensions of the internal dynamics and the specific knowledge and skills to build a cohesive team among the key players can dramatically improve the internal environment. At St Christoper's the key environmental factors were external politics and upward relationships. A greater insight into and influence on these dynamics might have averted the situation, and might well have protected Dr Roberts's position.

So why bother with management?

Doctors currently have the opportunity to have a full and active role in management, and it is vital for the future health of our hospitals and other health care organisations that this culture is maintained by clinicians taking up the challenge. Because hospitals and other provider units are complex to manage, the highest calibre and best informed management is required. Clinical professionals in all disciplines must play their part in demanding high calibre management - but must also be prepared themselves to make a significant and high quality contribution to management processes. The role of the doctor in management is to ensure that we "do things right, and do the right things." Doctors should play an active part in management not because it is the current fashion, or because "it is their turn" but because, for the benefit of patients, it is essential that the finite resources of the NHS must be invested on the basis of informed decision making. Without active involvement from clinicians in the management process poor decisions will continue to be taken, damaging organisations and patient care, just as they did at St Christopher's.

Key point summary

- Doctors must be involved in management decisions to influence the strategy of their organisation, and, therefore, the interests of their patients
- A single decision making body should be in place in every health care organisation, comprising significant numbers of doctors and managers, at which every major decision concerning the organisation is made
- Doctors' skills acquired in clinical practice can be used as a framework for management practice
- The complexities of hospital infrastructures and the demands imposed by the NHS reforms require highly developed management skills and appropriate management style, on the part of managers and doctors
- Explicit information based systems and team work are vital components of a decentralised management structure

---

1 NHS management inquiry. *Report.* (Griffiths report) London: DHSS, 1983.
2 Peters T, Austin N. *A passion for excellence.* London: Collins, 1986: 263.
3 Handy C. *The age of unreason.* Arrow, 1985: 106.
4 Mintzberg H. The professional context in the strategy process In: *Concepts, contexts and cases,* New York: Prentice-Hall Inc, 1988: 638–49.
5 Bamm, BMA, IHSM, RLN. *Managing clinical services.* London: Institute of Health Services Management, 1993.
6 Drucker P. *The effective executive.* London: Heinemann, 1986: 138–44.

2 Getting started as a medical manager

J F RIORDAN, JENNY SIMPSON

Case study

Three years after his appointment as a consultant physician Dr B was persuaded by his colleagues to become chairman of the cogwheel division of medicine, all the other physicians having taken their turn. He coped easily with running the monthly divisional meeting, found some satisfaction in juggling the junior medical rotas, and saw his most challenging role as resisting the attempts of the surgeons to "protect" their beds.

After a year in post a keen new general manager was appointed to take the hospital into trust status; he selected Dr B with several other consultants, not all of whom were divisional chairs, to form a management board. Dr B became the first clinical director of medicine. Initially he found this difficult as his colleagues continued to run the old divisional structure in parallel with the new arrangements. Also the senior nurses in medicine were suspicious of medical involvement in their management.

After some months of regular meetings with the nurse manager, along with several training and team building sessions, Dr B found that by working as part of a team he could influence the functioning of the medical service and achieved a number of successes. These included improving the process of case note retrieval; rearranging the appointments procedure; and developing a number of enthusiastic teams to take on specific projects within the directorate. After a few months the atmosphere and communication within the directorate had improved considerably, with staff of all grades beginning to contribute their ideas and support for the new systems. On the strength of this, Dr B managed to persuade his consultant colleagues to disband the cogwheel division and set up a full directorate structure with a number of subdirectorates. To his surprise he found that he enjoyed working with some of the newly recruited, bright, and keen business managers and took the opportunity to learn and develop new skills in negotiation, information management, time management, and financial monitoring and planning.

Now, with Dr B's three year fixed term period of directorship coming to an end and the hospital well established as a trust, he has to give up his post—just when he feels he is beginning to make the most valuable contribution. Having invested time and effort into organising the directorate and understanding its functioning, Dr B is determined that it should succeed. Fortunately, a capable deputy to Dr B had been appointed and trained over the past year, and Dr B has the satisfaction of knowing that she will continue the good work.

However, Dr B's interest in management has been stimulated and he is at present discussing with the chief executive his wish to take on further management responsibility. He will probably take a lead role in coordinating management development within the trust, which has declared as one of its objectives the decentralisation of clinical management down to subunit level. The chief executive has also asked him to become the trust's medical director. Other possibilities include involvement with a region wide training scheme for medical management, helping the medical school to develop an undergraduate course on management, and making a contribution to medical management at national level within the British Association of Medical Managers.

We live in times of constant change. There are increasing pressures for the NHS to be more efficient, more effective, and more responsive, and these are now accepted throughout the NHS.

The old approach of administering a relatively fixed and unchanged system has given way to the introduction of the techniques of general management which allow organisations to respond appropriately to change. The introduction of general management began with the Griffiths report of 1983 and has been continued since with the introduction of resource management, followed by the white paper *Working for Patients*, with its separation of the purchaser and provider functions. Inherent in all these changes has been the idea that doctors should have a pivotal role in managing health service resources.

Under the old system hospitals were organised into a series of separate hierarchies, functioning in semi-independent fashion. The system was resistant to change. The position of divisional chairman was often filled, on the "Buggin's turn" principle, by doctors who regarded the post as a tedious, but necessary chore.

With the introduction and subsequent dissemination of the resource management initiative in 1986-92 there was a major move towards integrating the various professional hierarchies into devolved directorate teams, giving individual clinical services the ability to respond flexibly to change in a coherent manner. These new structures have required doctors to take part in influencing the way in which care is delivered and in setting the future direction of the hospital. Many of those who have taken up the challenge have found it a rewarding experience, although there can be tensions between clinical practice and management.

Doctors who are not involved increasingly risk being managed by others and having less influence than at present, while those who accept directorate roles with the older divisional model in mind are likely to find themselves frustrated and disillusioned. All doctors need to understand the role of management and should contribute to it.

Making a start

Having decided to take management seriously the aspirant doctor–manager's first step should be to take an honest and critical look at his or her strengths and identify the weak spots. The knowledge of the totality of management, "what there is to know," and one's personal ability to get things done need cool appraisal. In the course of clinical training and practice many doctors will have acquired much knowledge and experience which is directly applicable to medical management. Normal clinical practice and medical audit bring familiarity with measuring activity, clinical coding, case mix, and aspects of quality. Organising junior doctors' rotas and training confer some knowledge of personnel issues.

On the other hand, many hospital doctors find themselves ignorant of the financial and accounting aspects of medical practice. Areas such as marketing, planning, and strategy may also feel alien, as do some of the broader issues of quality assurance and personnel management.

As well as assessing their knowledge of management issues doctors should also assess their management style and skills. Many very expert clinicians are rather less expert in communica-

---

Where to get help

Unit level
Organisational development manager
Training manager
Human resources manager
Medical director
Chief executive

Regional level
Resource coordinator for doctors in management
Regional management coordinator
Coordinator for medical audit
Regional postgraduate dean
Provider development department

National level
British Association of Medical Managers
British Medical Association
Institute of Health Services Management
National Association of Health Authorities and Trusts

Sources of funding
Study leave budget
Local or regional training budget
Sponsorship by pharmaceutical firms, etc

---

tion and negotiation, and few have understanding of, or training in, leadership skills or working in teams.

Help with this initial assessment can be obtained either locally in the hospital or sought further afield (box). The assessment may vary from informal, personal advice at hospital level to a much more formal and structured session at a management assessment centre. Further advice will then be required to set up a training programme. If starting from little or no management knowledge by far the most effective approach is to enrol on an introductory management course. This may be tailored specifically to doctors and run by the NHS in conjunction with organisations such as business schools. Such an initial course provides a good introduction to the subject and identifies areas where further training may be required. Following this, specific training needs should be addressed. Many suitable courses, seminars, and conferences are run by individual trusts, business schools, health services management units, and other national management

Business plan

(1) Service description
Activity
Case mix
Numbers
Sources of referrals

Staffing
Resources used
Buildings
Equipment
Non-pay items
Other services used

Monitoring and communication
Information systems
Management structure
Marketing
Quality and audit

Finance (based on all the above)
Income/expenditure
Capital charges
Balance sheet

(2) Goals and objectives

Mission statement
Objectives
Achievable
Measurable
Monitored
Set time scale

(3) Action plan (to achieve objectives)

New developments
Restrictions
Financial forecasts
How monitored

organisations. These are advertised in the health management press and in newsletters and other publications from the national associations (the Institute of Health Services Management, National Association of Health Authorities and Trusts, British Association of Medical Managers) and increasingly in the medical press.

While most doctors still equate management with the financial aspects (and a basic knowledge of these is undoubtedly important), most doctors will benefit more from undertaking some training in interpersonal and influencing skills. This is necessary to understand the modern view of management as an enabling and team based process, as opposed to the hierarchical, control based view still unfortunately fostered by the more traditional medical schools. In future these skills should be taught as an essential part of the undergraduate curriculum, as is just beginning to happen in the more enlightened schools.

Nevertheless, as in many areas of medicine, there is no substitute for learning by doing, and active experience should be sought from the beginning. All doctors can and should take some part in management in the course of their clinical training. Junior doctors can start through medical or preferably multi-disciplinary audit. Action resulting from the audit process translates into management at the departmental or unit level for all grades of medical staff. The doctor should take an interest in the management of his or her clinical directorate by attending directorate meetings and by being prepared to take part in the various management tasks involved in running the directorate—ask to see information, contribute ideas, and comments.

The senior registrar looking for a consultant post should include the management arrangements in any assessment of hospital posts and should think twice before applying to hospitals where medical staff talk of "administrators" and where there is a "them and us" culture. Instead, doctors should look for hospitals where clinicians are active in management and where there is a commitment to devolving management down to clinical subunits. Doctors in these organisations stand a much better chance of enjoying both a clinically rewarding career and a key role in influencing the direction in which the hospital develops.

How to get involved: the business plan

One of the best ways of playing an active part in management is to take part in drawing up the business plan. This process encompasses all aspects of the directorate and provides a valuable insight into the workings of the organisation. It may sound boring, but the business plan is now a mandatory part of the management of hospitals and directorates and can be applied throughout an organisation down to the smallest unit, ward, or laboratory. Even if business planning is not part of your organisation's culture, it is a worthwhile exercise at departmental level, among immediate colleagues.

The business plan

In essence the business plan sets out to answer three questions:
- Where are we now?
- Where do we want to go?
- How do we get there?

An assessment of the current state of the unit or department is carried out in terms of: workload, staffing, use of capital and non-pay items, methods of information gathering, and financial position in terms of income and expenditure. Then a range of clear and achievable objectives are agreed. The plan then defines how these are to be achieved and how progress is to be monitored with fallback plans for implementation if objectives are not being met.

While financial input is essential for the finalisation of the plan much ground work can be done before the finance department is involved. Accountants appreciate dealing with a directorate that knows its business and has a clear idea of where it wants to go. Having produced a business plan for the specialty or department, it is important to feed it into the planning process for the organisation as a whole and to be prepared to modify the plan if it conflicts with the overall business plan.

What is the downside of a managerial role?

An involvement in management demands that the doctor accepts responsibility for matters which could previously be left to others. Sometimes difficult decisions have to be made, which make the doctor–manager less than popular with his or her colleagues. This may have consequences rather more far reaching than temporary ill feeling and resentment, jeopardising relationships that hitherto may have been good. Some doctors report that they are now less than likely to be awarded higher merit awards, having unwittingly crossed swords with those with power and influence on the awarding bodies.

There are undoubtedly extra claims on the doctor's time, and further difficult decisions may have to be made between clinical and management demands. This can to some extent be less of a problem if the doctor can delegate responsibility. In taking on any management post it is important to make sure that there is someone of the appropriate skills and experience to whom work may be delegated. If this is not the case it should be an essential condition to taking on the job. Many doctors find management work overwhelming, and all doctors should ensure that they are soundly trained in the techniques of time management and delegation before taking on full management responsibility.

Conflict with colleagues is also a potential problem, although if handled positively such conflicts can sometimes be turned around into a constructive debate, which in the long run works to the benefit of all concerned. Again, there are management techniques to help with such situations, which can easily be acquired by the interested and committed doctor.

Far more difficult to overcome, however, is the risk of professional isolation, particularly if the medical management culture in the hospital is not strong. Clinical colleagues may regard the doctor–manager as colluding with the enemy. On the other hand, non-medical managers who see doctors as a threat to the management process are unlikely to welcome them with open arms. The doctor in management holds a lonely role in some of today's hospitals. Those who have taken this route have found that it is invaluable to have access to other medical colleagues involved in management, for exchanging ideas and information and for mutual support. If at all possible doctors–managers should build these relationships within their own institutions, and they may also find it helpful to join regional groups and national associations.

What are the rewards?

By far the most important reward of playing a part in management is the opportunity to work on the broader canvas of the organisation as a whole and to have a major influence on the development of a better service for patients. This is the major reward cited by clinical and medical directors, and many find the transition back to being non-managerial difficult. Indeed, some hospitals have developed other managerial roles for former clinical directors, so that their hard earned experience and skill is not wasted.

In future management input will probably increasingly be rewarded financially. At present some doctor–managers get extra sessional payments, some get extra clinical support, and some get extra paid leave. Management input is now also one factor considered during the asesssment procedure for C distinction awards. However, medical and clinical directors generally believe that the fundamental reward is likely to remain the professional satisfaction obtained from functioning as an effective member of a team having a major influence on the future direction and development of the clinical service.

Key point summary

- Much of the current training for medical students still prepares them for hierarchical, control based structures, and does not equip them for a team based process

- Many doctors lack communication and negotiation skills. They also have a poor understanding of, and little training in, leadership skills and team work

- Introductory management skills courses, training in time management, followed up by specific training courses run by one of the national management organisations, can make good these deficits

- Hands-on experience is needed: one of the best ways of getting started is to get involved in the directorate's business plan

- Despite the inevitable tensions between clinical practice and management, the extra time commitment, the need to make unpopular decisions and the resultant feelings of isolation, management can be fun, stimulating, and rewarding

3 Effective top teams: luxury or necessity?

ANDREW KAKABADSE, HUGH SMYLLIE

Case study

At a Medical Advisory Committee meeting in 1987 the consultant in accident and emergency proposed that in the light of a recent report by the Royal College of Physicians criticising the standard of cardiopulmonary resuscitation (CPR) in hospitals,[1] our district general hospital should review its training and procedures in CPR. The meeting agreed to form a subcommittee under the aegis of the consultant anaesthetist in charge of the intensive therapy unit. Other members were to be the proposer, the consultant responsible for coronary care unit, that unit's sister in charge, and a junior doctor. Also included was the senior operating department assistant because he and his colleagues were important members of the crash team bringing the crash trolley and performing intubation. The subcommittee chairman obtained advice from a regional cardiac centre who had already revised their CPR training and procedures.

The subcommittee duly met. Its members were defensive of their various roles and departments, there was an acrimonious clash of personalities between consultants, and the meeting broke up having achieved nothing.

No further attempt was made to pursue the issue until 1991, by which time the district general hospital had become an NHS trust. One of the trust's early decisions was to develop a resuscitation policy to include procedures and training. The task was allocated to the medical director who delegated it to the clinical director of anaesthetics whose directorate included operating theatres. This anaesthetist became the chair of a new working party on CPR. He was advised to limit the working party to four consultants, two of whom were on the previous subcommittee. He was also advised to seek opinions from relevant experts within and, if necessary, outside the hospital.

Initially, he approached members and experts individually to indicate those aspects on which they should contribute a brief written submission. He amalgamated these into a draft report which was circulated in advance of the working party's meeting. At that meeting, each member was encouraged to comment on the report in general and to the section relating to their own special interest. Members were guided back to their remit if they digressed inappropriately. Agreement on the framework of a final draft was reached in just over one hour. The trust now has a modern resuscitation policy with built in outcome review.

Learning points

Team failure

In 1987 the failure of the team was due to:

- the formation of the team as a result of the reactive response of the Medical Advisory Committe rather than a proactive initiative;
- the lack of clear mandate or direct recommendations to the team;
- the inability to lead the team from a corporate perspective, so that although the team was composed of all the relevant internal experts, the players concerned ended up defending their departments and traditional roles in terms of providing a resuscitation service;
- lack of preparedness which included no objective advice being offered to the chair. He could therefore incorporate only those aspects that suited his viewpoint, thus creating a suspicion of bias;
- the individualistic nature of the key players, especially the consultants, which led to an uncomfortable clash of personalities.

Team success

In 1992 the more successful impact made by the team was due to:

- a clear proactive decision taken by the trust, subject to internal market forces, to provide for a quality resuscitation service;
- the effectiveness and authority of the team in terms of its size and cohesion by having only four senior consultants;
- the advice received by the chair, this time focusing on procedure, principally in terms of calling on other expertise such as resuscitation staff from all levels;

- greater ownership of the project, with members of the team producing written submissions;
- the overall effectiveness of meetings, because of good preparation, prior communication of draft documents, and firm but sympathetic adherence to the agenda.

Is the situation outlined in 1987 in the case study example untypical of the NHS, or more broadly, of organisations from both the private and public sectors? The answer is an emphatic no. Extensive survey work shows the norm is that uncomfortable team dynamics and considerably ineffective behaviour at the top of the organisation is prevalent not only in Britain, but also in senior executives from most other European countries (box).[2]

That does not alter the fact that teams are vital. Without effective top teams an organisation cannot function efficiently. Teams are the prime mechanism for both the consideration and implementation of policies and strategies. Senior executives need a forum in which to discuss the fundamental issues that face the organisation, and identify and agree to implement approaches that will address current and future concerns and challenges.

However, if the members of the top management group feel that the quality of relationships, the ability to reach decisions, the commitment to the decisions reached and the will to implement the decisions made is lacking, then unfortunately there will be a gulf between what ought to happen and what actually does

---

Trends from the Cranfield Executive Development Survey in the United Kingdom and Ireland

- 40% of general managers feel negative about their senior bosses in the senior team

- 58% of chairs, chief executive officers, and managing directors feel uncomfortable about the effectiveness of the senior team and the performance of its members

- 51% of chief executive officers, managing directors, and General Managers feel there are important and sensitive issues at top level which remain unaddressed

- 63% of senior management recognise that there are substantial hindrances to achieving objectives in the senior team

happen. If the quality of dialogue among the members of the senior executive is more negative or overly sensitive then the issues facing the team and the organisation may be only too well understood by the members of the senior team, but their relationships will be so strained that concerns about the organisation (and potential solutions to problems) may be unable to surface, because the discomfort generated in doing so would be too much for any one of them to bear. This makes for a bad and ineffective team.

Shaping the team

Shaping the team is critical to shaping the future, and not only involves understanding and appropriately shaping a potentially demanding and disparate group of people into a cohesive whole, but also recognising how the top team directly affects the overall business.

To create an effective team at the top is entirely in the hands of the members of the top management of the organisation. Five factors should be considered:

- a need for a key forum for dialogue;
- each member of the team needs to get on well with one another;
- positive executive relationships;
- the way issues, be they sensitive or not, are addressed;
- effective management styles and philosophy.

The difference between an effective and ineffective team is not that a fundamental compatibility exists among its members, but that serious consideration has been given as to how the personalities in the senior team interrelate. In an effective team attempts have been made to create an environment conducive to generating a meaningful discussion about the business. This may involve inducing a certain amount of tension in the group, but not to the point where it undermines cohesion. The 1991 attempt to improve the CPR standard in the case study involved generating a far more positive dialogue, in terms of preparation for meetings, documentation, and honest and open conversation.

Those executives who do not seriously consider the impact of the interrelationships of the personalities on the top team are also not likely to have thought about the impact they themselves make on the group in terms of stimulating positive relationships, or in creating an open culture. They also tend to just react to their colleagues on the team. The ones who have considered their

31

impact on their team colleagues have attempted seriously to adjust their approach to adopt both a style and a philosophy conducive to the team and the business.

Meaningful research

What, then, is required for health service organisations in terms of senior management performance, especially now that forces such as internal markets have been created? The question that needs to be addressed is what needs to be done to make health service structures perform more effectively?

Consideration needs to be given to the following areas of research:

- executive competency of the key senior executive roles represented on the NHS trust boards;
- the effectiveness of the newly established structures, how the key internal interfaces are being managed, and whether those issues and concerns are being addressed, and the subsequent impact on quality of service provision;
- the external interface between regional health authorities, district health authorities, and general practitioner fundholders, and their impact on the management and effective service delivery of trusts.

Effective decision making

Understanding the quality of dialogue at both key internal and external interfaces within NHS trusts will provide valuable clues as to the effectiveness of decision making and implementation of policy. If a continuum were to be drawn which identified the key influences on decision making, at one end would be logic and at the other end emotions and personalities (fig 3.1)

Decisions based on logic identify business and economic trends using data. A process of extrapolation allows decisions to be made. The interplay of personalities at the senior management levels means that decisions are driven by emotions. Who influences who, who was the last one to see the boss after the meeting, and the overall mix of chemistries between personalities can all seriously influence the nature of the decisions made and the way in which they are implemented.

A full appreciation of the nature of the internal markets and the qualities required of senior management to address sensitive internal and external interfaces, and the desired dynamics of

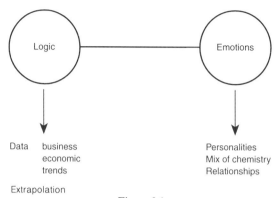

Figure 3.1

effective top teams, means that the effective senior manager should be able to reach a balanced view. In other words open dialogue about the business and awareness of the personalities and relationships concerned, to ensure that commitment on decisions is reached, so providing the basis for actioning the insights and expertise already in existence within the senior team. Without it the potential of staff and management could be seriously compromised. The question is, will senior management teams rise to the challenge?

Key point summary

- Teams are an essential component of the new organisational structure

- Relationships between key personalities can make or break a team: an understanding of these dynamics is imperative

- Teams often fail because they lack a clear mandate and a corporate perspective

- Teams succeed when they are proactive, well prepared, and communicate well

- It is essential that a forum for open and frank discussion is actively promoted

- A team's effectiveness needs to be regularly assessed

1 Report of the Royal College of Physicians. Resuscitation from Cardiopulmonary arrest — training and organisation. *J R Coll Physicians Lond* 1987; **21**: 175-82.
2 Kakabadse A. *Wealth creators*. London: Kogan Page, 1992.

4 Conflict, power, negotiation

LIAM DONALDSON

Conflict, how it arises and how it is resolved, is closely related to where power lies within a hospital, health authority, or medical practice and how this is influenced by external factors. This is a subtle and complex process which differs enormously from one health care organisation to another, over time, and from issue to issue. Power can influence change in predictable and conventional ways. For example, in the choice of a new member of the medical staff of a hospital, the head of the relevant clinical department and his or her consultant colleagues are likely to be the principal determinants of the type of individual chosen. On the other hand, a major and unforeseen impact on the organisation might be produced by a quite junior member of staff whose power derives from the possession of information which could be passed anonymously to local media and arouse public concern.

Conflict exists whenever individual or group interests diverge within an organisation, and if its values or goals are at odds with those of the external environment. These considerations apply to the operation of both private and public sector enterprises, but, in the latter, the influence of the wider public and political dimension makes the process of setting and achieving objectives in an orderly way much more complex. In health care organisations the potential for conflict arising through internal and external factors is ever present. The resolution of such conflict is often the route to progress or the way in which major change takes place. It is one of the jobs of management to understand the potential sources of conflict and to be able to predict how, when, and why they will arise. Similarly, effective management of change is not possible without a clear understanding of the sources of power within the organisation and how they can be harnessed, not just to resolve conflict, but to bring about improvement and generate innovation.

The NHS reforms in 1990 introduced new mechanisms for the organisation and funding of health care in Britain.[1] By separating the responsibility for purchasing care from that for its provision, these reforms sought to reorientate the management of the service by changing the role of existing organisations. The functioning of the reorganised health service now depends on the interaction between bodies that purchase health care for populations (health authorities and fundholding practices) and those which provide it (mainly NHS trust hospitals and community service units). This system of public health care provision introduced new forces which were intended to produce better and more efficiently provided services within an internal market.

Despite the creation of an environment which should make explicit the decisions about population needs for health care and how they are most appropriately to be met, many changes to the way in which health services are delivered are not based on a detached assessment of such factors. Instead, it is the interests and aspirations of hospitals as local institutions, of the senior staff working within them, and of the local community (including its general practitioners) which are often the driving force for change.

Change, and the threat or the possibility of it, produces uncertainty and can result in conflict. The role of management in these circumstances is to recognise the inevitability of change and to help the organisation (and the individuals within it) to deal with uncertainty whilst moving towards its overall goals. Uncertainty is not a source of power. Rather, it is coping with uncertainty which confers power.[2] Management's credibility and thus its effectiveness are greatly increased where it can introduce stability and clarity of direction in situations of rapid change or conflict.

Case study

Sidebridge, a metropolitan area with a population of some 200 000, has traditionally looked to the neighbouring teaching hospital, St George's, rather than its local general hospital for a range of its specialist health care services. From being a hospital with an undistinguished clinical reputation, one which did not attract strong fields of applicants for new consultant posts, and which was not recognised for postgraduate training in many specialties, Sidebridge General Hospital has been transformed over the past 20 years. The unit general manager, Nathan Crossthwaite, has spent his whole career in Sidebridge, having worked his way up the hospital administration ladder since leaving school. However, the driving force for these changes has been its senior surgeon, Arnold Nexus. He is a widely respected local figure and highly skilled medical politician who has demonstrated repeatedly his ability to influence health service planning committees, lead large and successful charitable fund raising appeals, and receive highly favourable coverage in the local media. As a result Sidebridge General Hospital has received the largest level of capital investment in buildings and equipment of any comparable hospital in the country; it had the first magnetic resonance imaging (MRI) scanner outside a teaching centre and has won the Citizen's Chartermark for the quality of its diabetes service.

Before his retirement, Nexus is determined to see a specialist ear nose and throat (ENT) surgery service established locally in Sidebridge to rival that in the teaching hospital of St George's. In his attempts to develop services in the hospital he has been frustrated by the professor of surgery at St George's, Harold Rostrevor (with whom he was at medical school). Rostrevor has repeatedly attempted to block progress, using his role as the university representative on consultant appointment committees to veto locally favoured candidates, and by refusing to sanction a senior registrar rotation encompassing Sidebridge. Nexus is also convinced that Rostrevor has held back his preferment in the distinction awards system.

Plans for a local ENT surgery service were finally driven through but implementation was beset by problems from the outset. The recruitment of consultants proved difficult because potential applicants made adverse comparisons with the St George's department. However, eventually two consultants were recruited and the local service started. General practitioners' views on the development of the local service had not been explicitly sought. They began to refer minor cases to the new Sidebridge service but most of their referrals continued to flow to St George's. Within a year, it was obvious that the new local service was seriously underused.

The NHS reforms seemed to offer a way out of the impasse in that the Sidebridge District Health Authority intended to place the ENT surgery service contract with the local general hospital. The ENT surgery situation was exacerbated when six months later four of Sidebridge's general practices became fundholders and started openly discussing terminating their contracts with the general hospital based service in favour of that at St George's. Alarmed by this potential shift in contracts, the district health authority (which as the sole remaining purchaser of the local service would have been adversely affected by the fundholder withdrawal) started urgent discussions with Sidebridge's general practitioners regarding their referral preferences for ENT surgery work.

Following these discussions with both fundholding and non-fundholding general practices, district health authority managers decided to shift all ENT surgery work from Sidebridge to St George's. Their decision was made public at a meeting of the health authority. At this point, the local media, which until then had taken only a passing interest in the discussions concerning the future of the ENT surgery service at Sidebridge, became involved following their receipt of a petition signed by 45 nurses and junior doctors decrying the proposed contract shift as a cutback in local services. Over the next two months a campaign in the local press drew in both local councillors and the Sidebridge Community Health Council.

The situation was brought under control when the new chief executive of the Sidebridge Hospital NHS Trust, Gary Masters, persuaded the general manager of the district health authority and the chief executive of the St George's Trust to agree to a review of the service. A senior ENT surgical consultant from outside the area was asked to lead a visiting team which examined data on morbidity, referral patterns, waiting times and contract prices. They held a series of meetings with all interested individuals and groups. A report was produced which recommended the consolidation of ENT surgery services at the St George's site but with transfer of all Sidebridge staff (including the two consultants). These recommendations were accepted and it was agreed that the changes would be phased in over two years.

Analysis of issues in the case study

The case study depicts a situation in which the personal vision of a charismatic senior doctor becomes intertwined with his hospital's aspirations. It encompasses many of the issues and decisions which are pivotal to the modern NHS. How many hospitals can a large urban conurbation sustain? What types of services should they provide? What is a "specialist" service and how should it be delivered? Does the internal market created by the reforms mean that hospitals should compete flat out, or generally cooperate in ensuring that the population receives the service that it needs?

Sources of conflict

The events described arise from sources of conflict which will be very familiar to those working within the health service: the single mindedness of one respected individual; major interpersonal conflict between two senior doctors; years of power play and rivalry between a teaching hospital and its general hospital neighbour; assumptions that general practitioners will simply fit in with service changes which affect them; and the tendency of the local media to simplify complex issues in a way which heightens public concern.

The surgeon at Sidebridge held power not by virtue of his formal authority but through his ability to build up strong networks and constituencies which would support him when key decisions were made about the allocation of resources to his hospital. His command of public opinion through his fund raising work and his use of local media to promote the hospital, gave him a further power base through which to influence at a number of levels. It has not been unusual in the past for a single doctor to be the dominant force in an institution and, in effect, as here, to set the strategic direction for a hospital. Power approaches to organisational theory[3-5] directly challenge earlier models of how organisations make decisions which emphasised rationality. A large number of sources have been identified through which power is derived within organisations. Some of the main ones are shown in the box.

The underlying forces which led to power being exercised to produce change were complex. They included Sidebridge Hospital's sense of institutional pride, a desire to place local access considerations above those of economies of scale and potentially better outcomes, and a longstanding rivalry between the hospital and its more prestigious neighbour. The seeds of change were also sown by the personal animosity between two influential individuals and a sense of injustice on the part of one of them.

Hospital management style

The role of hospital management was initially subordinate to the part played by the doctors. Too often hospital management has found itself at one or other end of a spectrum of control. Either it has remained remote and distant from doctors and other senior professional staff in the hospital, taking decisions in isolation and then expecting them to be understood and implemented enthusiastically as well as effectively. Or management has seen itself as there simply to support the actions of senior doctors in the hospital. In the case study the unit general manager fell into the latter category. Some managers who entered the health service in the 1950s and 1960s, when traditional values and power relationships meant that the role of management ("administration" as it was referred to then) was, at best, facilitation, have also tended to behave in this way.

This style of management is not entirely a feature of some older managers. The rapid growth of managerial posts in the late 1980s and early 1990s means that many relatively young people hold senior managerial posts. A small proportion have neither the maturity, interpersonal skills, nor formal management training to lead a workforce of strong willed, highly educated, senior professional staff. On several occasions, I have visited hospitals where the senior manager has privately admitted that he or she is in effect "frightened" of the consultants. This invariably leads to conflict either inside the institution, because the senior manager adopts an autocratic style of mangement, or outside, because the hospital moves in a direction which is not in keeping with the needs of the service.

Personalities

Aside from the balance of power between management and hospital doctors in Sidebridge, a further factor which produced conflict was the tension between the clinical academic service and the health service. This conflict was evident both at the individual and the institutional level. One of the great strengths of the NHS is the generally close partnership between the academic and service components in the delivery of patient care, in postgraduate training, and in research. Sometimes things go wrong in these relationships and when they do it usually concerns two factors: disputes over territory; and the inappropriate use of power. Both were evident in the example described. The conflict between the professor of surgery and the local surgeon went beyond mere professional rivalry and was exacerbated by the professor's possession of power based on his formal authority (consultant appointments), his command of networks (ability to influence), and his control over scarce resources (distinction awards, training posts) (box). This somewhat despotic behaviour is fortunately rare but when it does occur it can be ingrained and difficult to resolve.

Sources of power within organisations

- Holding formal authority
- Controlling scarce resources
- Having information
- Possessing special expertise
- Displaying the ability to cope with uncertainty
- Commanding strong networks
- Belonging to the dominant culture

Diverging philosophies and the resolution of conflict

The demands brought about by the reforms generated additional conflict in Sidebridge. The imperative explicitly to match service requirements to population need and efficient use of resources threw serious doubt on the decision to create a local ear, nose, and throat (ENT) surgery service. The strengthened role of general practice (both generally and specifically through the fundholding scheme) introduced a further dimension. Moreover, the need for hospitals which became NHS trusts to produce a clear statement of their strategic direction also contributed to the burgeoning local crisis.

Public perceptions

The prospect of change generated immediate and major conflict within the communities affected, among staff in the hospitals concerned, and in other local agencies and organisations. In the public's mind the justification for change was not understood or simply just not accepted. The management of the NHS persistently fails to capture the widespread support of the public for its policies. Decisions based on considerations of improved outcome of clinical care or better use of resources can lead to rationalisation of services delivered by particular hospital departments. Such events are then construed by the public as failures of the system rather than the inevitable consequence of a continual improvement in the quality of care, aided and abetted by innovation in medical science, in a service striving to maximise limited resources.

Doctors and other health care professionals have considerable power to generate conflict and affect the process of change by shaping public attitudes and beliefs through their use of the media (the petition in this example). This is so even if the individuals are not representative of the views of their peer group.

The need for impartiality

The new chief executive of the local hospital as it became an NHS trust was the person who took the initiative to resolve the conflict. He recognised that the solution could come only through negotiation and mediation. In such situations people usually recognise that conflict, an impasse, or a crisis must be resolved if public confidence in the service is to be restored. Their expectation is not necessarily for a compromise which satisfies all points of view, but more that the evidence should be examined objectively, that all relevant voices should be heard, and that a decision should be based fairly on both (fig 4.1).

A review carried out quickly by a person of standing from outside the area is an excellent approach and one which is increasingly frequently being used in the modern health service when such serious conflicts arise. The person coming in from outside, if chosen correctly, is seen as impartial and can fulfil a role which those directly involved cannot because of fears about their motivation. People do not necessarily expect a happy ending to a controversial situation like the one described, but they do expect the outcome to be a return to stability.

Lessons for the future

Too often strategic decisions are characterised by the identification of a desired end point, but a failure to persuade people of the need for the change or to take them along with the process. Successful delivery of a strategy requires the calibre of management to provide skilled negotiation and leadership to persuade all interest groups of the importance of change and to inspire them that the end result is worth achieving (fig 4.2). This is particularly so for the dominant culture, the clinical one, with its powerful networks and high public credibility.

Conclusions

In the late 1980s it was recognised that hospitals would be

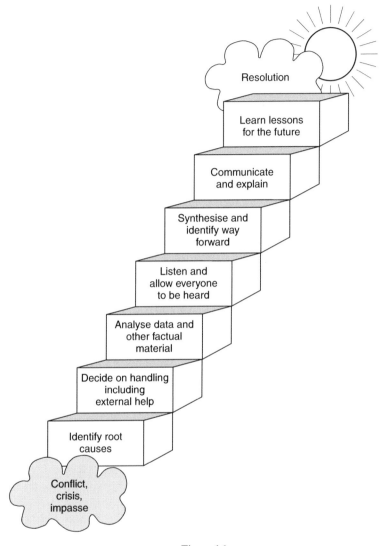

Figure 4.1

much more effective organisations if doctors were more directly involved in the management process. This led to the growth in the availability of performance and financial information for clinicians and to the creation of medical management posts at hospital level,

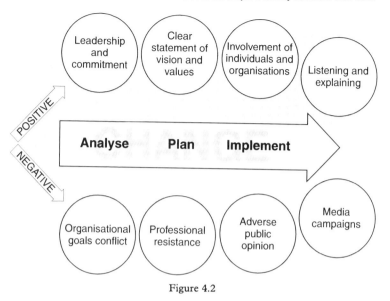

Figure 4.2

clinical directors of service departments, and more recently medical directors on NHS trust hospital boards.

The health service of the 1990s faces major strategic decisions: determining the balance between primary, secondary, and community care on a population basis; examining the centrality of the traditional general hospital in the health care system; and anticipating major technological change. Increasingly as hospitals and health authorities regularly and formally review their current roles and future aspirations, management will have to do much more than manage the operational level of service. In this challenging environment the service will need not only the best of managers but also more extensive involvement of doctors in the strategic management process. These doctors will have the complex task of sharing in difficult, sometimes deeply unpopular decisions, and of subordinating their institutional or professional loyalties to wider health goals. As part of this process they may find themselves discharging a special role in influencing and persuading their peers and in explaining the changes to the media and the general public.

An understanding of the likely points of conflict when change is heralded, the sources of power within health care organisations and systems, and the way in which they are resolved or harnessed will be just some of the management skills needed by doctors in the future.

Key point summary

- Conflict can arise from a clash of powerful personalities, uncertainty in the face of change, and management versus clinical considerations

- Effective management hinges on knowledge of the sources of power in an organisation and how these might conflict, and persuading people of the need for change and involving them in the process

- Negotiation and mediation are central to the resolution of conflict; and sometimes in a crisis, this is best undertaken by an impartial "outsider"

- Doctors need to become more involved in management decisions and process to have an effective role and an understanding of management needs

---

1 *National Health Service and Community Care Act 1990*. London: HMSO, 1990.
2 Hickson DJ, Hinings CR, Lee CA, Schneck RE, Pennings JM. A strategic contingencies theory of intra-organisational power. *Administrative Science Quarterly* 1971; **16**: 216–29.
3 Emerson RM. Power-dependence relations. *American Sociological Review* 1962: 27: 31–41.
4 Pettigrew AM. *The politics of organisational decision-making*. London: Tavistock Institute, 1973.
5 Pfeffer J. *Power in organisations*. Boston, Massachusetts: Pitman, 1981.

5 Managing change

PETER C BARNES

Case study : rationalisation of hospital services

Henford General Hospitals Trust comprises a large teaching hospital, Henford General, on the periphery of the former district and a small hospital, Saint Judes, in a deprived inner city area. Saint Judes has served the local population well for over 100 years and has gained an excellent reputation.

Considerable opposition was mounted, unsuccessfully, to the closure of its Accident and Emergency Department several years ago, to centralise the services on a single site at the main hospital. It has been understood for some time that a substantial development at Henford General would, at some stage, lead to the transfer of all services from Saint Judes and its subsequent closure. As a result, planning blight has afflicted Saint Judes and staff morale has plummeted.

Henford General Hospitals Trust has recently undergone major management reorganisation, leading to the introduction of clinical directorates which have now been in existence for two years. Some very clear improvements in service have resulted from this development and the organisation as a whole has adjusted well to the cultural change. Nevertheless, the clinical directors still feel a conflict of loyalties between the needs of individual patients and the needs of the organisation as a whole, particularly when considering the difficult financial circumstances of the Trust. Many are disappointed that their successes with efficiency savings have not led to direct benefit to their own services. Escalating costs, continued cost improvement programmes, uncertainty about purchaser intentions and potential instability with regard to local fundholding general practitioners have all become part of the daily routine of the management and the Trust which is under considerable pressure to balance its books. The regional health authority plan for a shift of resources within the region using a weighted capitation formula shows that Henford District will be a relative loser and as a result will receive only the minimum increase in annual funding and have less growth money than in previous years. Although used to experiencing considerable financial difficulties, the feeling in the main hospital is that crisis point has now been reached.

Early in the present financial year it became clear that the unit was heading for a major overspend that was unlikely to be met by marginal savings within each directorate. A task group was set up to look at the feasibility of an early transfer of all services from Saint Judes to Henford General to permit the closure of Saint Judes and the realisation of recurring revenue savings. Before the task group had completed its report considerable opposition to the move was voiced by staff at Saint Judes led by two well respected clinicians, the Community Health Council, and members of the public who lobbied MPs and presented a petition objecting to the closure to the Health Secretary. Board members expressed anxiety that a premature closure of Saint Judes might lead to service reductions and jeopardise contract income and the future development of the Trust. Nevertheless, after consideration of the task group's report which indicated the feasibility of transfer with minimum effect on services, they reluctantly recommended the transfer of services by the end of the calendar year.

Analysis

In the case cited the dilemmas and pressures are obvious and, unfortunately, not unique to the NHS. In recommending the early closure of Saint Judes and endeavouring to deliver Henford's acute services from a single site, the management board has taken a decision fraught with potential problems. How to proceed depends on how mature and effective the decision making structures have become since the development of clinical directorates. Whatever the decision, it is unlikely to be one which will command universal approval. In this situation the vital thing is to secure a decision making and change process that is as open as possible. This will not guarantee success but will give better prospects. At least those involved should understand what is happening, and why.

An analysis of the situation can be made using a modified version of the Nadler and Tushman diagnostic model (fig 5.1).[1]

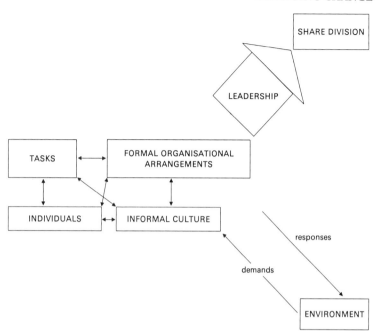

Figure 5.1 A model for organisational structure and function.

The organisation is seen as responding to, and in turn influencing, the external environment, and internally it is seen to comprise four components:

- the tasks
- the informal organisational arrangements
- the informal culture
- the individuals

The use of a such a model will not only allow organisational problems and the need for change to be analysed but will also help to identify areas of potential opposition to the intended changes.

People resist change for many reasons, but some of the most common are parochial self interest, misunderstanding and lack of trust, different assessments of the problems and solutions, and low tolerance for change.

Change and the tasks

The tasks are the activities which need to be carried out if the

47

organisation is to meet its goals. Current emphasis on objective setting in the NHS is highlighting the importance of this component which is the quantity and quality of service provided. It is to be expected that some opposition will be based on arguments about reductions in quantity or quality of service, or both, and it is important that honest and explicit statements are made about the expected impact of the transfer of services. Managers who initiate change often believe that they have all the relevant information required to conduct an adequate organisational analysis and also that those who will be affected by the change are fully aware of the facts. Neither assumption may be correct. Legitimate opposition based on more valid assessments should be given appropriate recognition.

Change and the formal structure

The formal organisational arrangements include accountability, job definition, pay structures, etc, and are usually fairly straightforward to describe. The reorganisation and new descriptions of these under the new arrangements is a fundamental management task which should be undertaken at the outset of the change process. While the period of turbulence is at its height and until a new set of organisational arrangements is in place, there may well be resistance which manifests itself in attempts to maintain control through the old formal mechanisms. An appeal from the medical staff committee at Saint Judes direct to the purchasing authority or the regional health authority would be an example of this.

Change and the informal culture

The informal culture is less tangible but more enduring than its formal counterpart and is often the life force of the organisation. The power bases of the organisation—who has what influence and why—are a fundamental part of the informal culture, which, at Saint Judes, will also embrace the long history and tradition of good service. Nevertheless, there has been planning blight and a reduction in staff morale. The informal culture will also include some degree of openness and readiness to change, and a willingness to maximise the benefits that will arise from a clear decision and the removal of uncertainty about the future.

Change and individuals

Individuals' reactions to change differ because of who they are, how they will be affected, and because their perceptions and knowledge about the change will vary. Medical and other staff may be worried about the dissolution of well established teams in theatre, others may have simpler concerns—for example, about transport difficulties and possible consequences on childminding arrangements. The changes may call for an adjustment in the numbers, skill mix, and experience of staff. Ensuring that individual needs are met in the new arrangements can be a major source of difficulty at times of rapid or enforced change.

Change and leadership

The model also shows the clear responsibility of senior management to shape, define, and encourage a shared vision of a better future, without which appropriate and successful change will not occur.

Managing the change

Having identified the problem, the need for change, and the intended solution, senior management need to make it happen. The following steps are minimum requirements in managing the change:

- Describing the future
- Publicising the change
- Commitment planning
- Action planning
- Maintaining the status quo

Describing the future

Given the legitimate anxiety of many people about the nature of the problem at Henford General Hospitals Trust and the perceived reduction in quantity and quality of service that may ensue, it is essential that these issues are clearly addressed with regard to each element of the diagnostic model. High priority should be given to concerns about patient care (the tasks), and what changes are likely in terms of numbers, skills, and attitude (the individuals). There should be a clear and coherent human resource strategy which takes into account opportunities for redeployment, retraining, and voluntary retirement. For example, redundancies could be minimised by vacancy control in the period before transfer, and the opportunities to form new and better teams should not be overlooked.

Publicising the change

As a result of the vocal opposition already mounted accurate and informed publicity is essential. Much will depend on the reliability and extent of information networks in the trust—for example, team briefing, newsletters, and staff meetings. People should be given information as soon as possible to minimise rumour and to allow them time to adjust.

Commitment planning

As well as developing the change strategy, the planner has to determine who in the organisation must be committed to the change if it is actually to take place. These key players are then assessed on a scale of commitment:

No commitment   likely to oppose the change
Let it happen   will not oppose the initiative but will not actively support it
Help it happen   must provide resources (time or equipment)
Make it happen   must be actively involved and willing to lead

The person's current position and where they need to be for the change to occur are charted on a table. The difference between the two is a crude measure of the work which may need to be done to obtain the necessary commitment from the key players (fig 5.2). In charting the person's position a degree of scepticism is sometimes necessary; expressed support is not always followed by appropriate action and sometimes covert resistance is encountered.

Action planning

The action plan is a list of all the tasks that will need to be completed for the change to take place. It is the road map of the change process. It is critical that it is realistic and effective. It should be relevant to the change goals, specific, integrated, time sequenced and adaptable. The task details, start and finish date, and responsible personnel should be published and circulated to all involved. In the case of the transfer of Saint Judes up to a 100 major separate tasks will probably need to be coordinated. This

Key players	No commitment	Let it happen	Help it happen	Make it happen
Chief executive officer				OX
Chairman St Judes medical staff committee	O →	X		
UMB member A		O →		X
UMB member B			O →	X
Consultant C		O → X		
Consultant D		X ←		O
Manager E		O →		X

O = present position; X = required position.
(Consultant D has poor interpersonal skills and his enthusiasm is likely to be counter-productive.

Figure 5.2 Commitment chart

will involve a large number of people and considerably stretch the organisation's resources.

Maintaining the status quo

The scale of the changes in Henford make it unlikely that the same volume of work could be accommodated during the change period. This should be explicitly stated so that everyone knows what standards are to be maintained. There can be a perceived status differential, with routine work being seen as less important than the change project, and therefore the support and encouragement of those who are keeping the hospital on target with its clinical work should be recognised and undertaken.

Coping with change

Success in change, particularly where professionals are concerned, turns on the ability to face real issues in an open enough manner to allow people to experience a sense of their own ability to influence their own destiny and to cope with the pressures and uncertainties inevitably generated by change. Individuals have four main categories of need amid a programme of organisational change. They need intelligible information. They will probably need to develop new skills, if only those needed to deal with new people as colleagues or supervisors. They will need support to help them deal with new problems. First and foremost, however, is a need for empathy. Pierre Casse defines empathy as follows:

"Empathy is the ability to see and understand how other people construct reality, or more specifically how they perceive, discover and invent the inner and outer worlds. We all use empathy. All the time. We constantly guess what people think and feel. The problem is that in most cases we guess wrongly. We assume that what is going on in somebody else's mind is somewhat identical to our own psychic processes. We tend to forget we are different. Sometimes drastically different. To practice empathy is to recognise and take full advantage of those differences."[2]

Conclusion

To manage changes effectively involves the ability to create a new synthesis of people, resources, ideas, opportunities and demands. The capacity to create systematic plans to provide for the logistics of resources, support, training and people is central to any programme of change. People must be influenced, departmental boundaries crossed or even "swallowed-up," new ideas must be accepted and new ways of working embraced. The politics of the organisation are crucial. Support must be mobilised, coalitions built, opposition handled and bargains struck. People will need help to cope with the stress, anxiety, and uncertainties of change. Continuity of tradition must be overturned, in part, as the old is replaced by the new. Yet continuity and tradition provide people with stability, support and meaning, and should not needlessly be destroyed. The effective management of organisational change demands the resolution of these apparently conflicting challenges.

The help of Colin Carnell is gratefully acknowledged.

1 Nadler Tushman. *Perspectives of behaviour*. New York: McGraw Hill, 1977.
2 Casse P. *Training for the cross-cultural mind*. Washington, DC: Society for Intercultural Education, Training and Research, 1979.

Key point summary

- The decision making and change processes should be as open as possible

- The tasks, the informal organisational arrangements, the informal culture and the individuals need to be analysed

- To make change happen effectively, it needs to be described clearly, publicised, committed to, action taken, and the status quo preserved

- The politics of the organisation are critical

- Foresight in terms of training needs is essential

- People's difficulties, when faced with change, should be respected, not ignored, and dealt with

- Continuity and tradition should not be destroyed just for the sake of it

6 Analysing your organisation and environment and setting its strategy

JOHN SM ZORAB, ANN LLOYD

Frenchay Healthcare Trust was a second wave trust and came into being on 1 April 1992. It has an annual budget of £89m and employs 4000 staff. The organisational structure, comprising seven clinical directorates and four executive directorates, was introduced the previous summer.

The underlying philosophy of the organisational structure is that the delivery of the clinical service is the responsibility of those consultants who have been appointed as clinical directors. The clinical directors are central to the management process and are directly accountable to the chief executive. This places the clinical directors firmly within a general management context

Frenchay Healthcare (NHS) Trust   **Trust board**
Chair and five non-executive members   plus

Chief executive	Medical director	Business director	Finance director	Chief nurse

Frenchay Healthcare (NHS) Trust management team						
Chief executive						
Director of surgery	Director of neuro-science	Director of clinical support	Director of clinical facilities	Director of mental health	Director of medicine	Director of community services
	Medical director	Business director	Chief nurse	Finance director	Personnel director	Operations director
chair, medical staff committee (co-opted)						

without any intervening tiers filtering the communication and accountability between them and the chief executive.

This, combined with the consequent responsibility that goes with budgetary control and the management of staff and contracts, has enabled the relevant consultants and managers to work as unitary teams. Responsibility for setting the direction for each directorate within the whole organisation truly rests with the clinical director—together with the management and coordination of directorate activities.

An essential component of this system is that each clinical director is supported by a high quality general manager (grade SMP 13-15) together with, in some instances, a I grade senior specialist clinical nurse. Nevertheless, both the general manager and the senior nurse are responsible to the clinical director for the work of the directorate. Thus the clinical director is not a medical manager but a director supported by a professional manager and a professional nurse.

All clinical directors sit on the management team, which advises the chief executive on all strategic, policy, and major operational issues. Clinical directors, therefore, influence decisions affecting the whole trust within which they must manage their directorates.

It is our firm belief that consultants do not need to learn to be professional managers. They do, however, have to learn the language and skills of their managerial role to function effectively as heads of specialty, clinical directors, or as medical directors. General managers also have had to learn to understand better the clinical perceptions of their clinical directors.

Strategic direction of the trust

This management structure, however, has to work within, and be able to pursue, the strategic direction of the trust, as set by the trust board in the light of advice from the management team. The mission statement of the trust incorporates the phrase: "Excellence in practice" and, at an early stage in the life of the trust, the trust board agreed that the strategic direction to be followed should be based on the following precepts.

The service provided would:

- respond to the needs of patients;
- by "excellence in practice", provide the highest possible quality of health care;
- respond to the needs of purchasers;
- play its part in the implementation and achievement of national strategies for healthcare.

The above precepts also indicate the agreed priorities. *Patients come first.*

The principles adopted by the management team to achieve this broad based strategy were:

- to build on the strengths of the organisation and its services;
- to analyse and, where appropriate, implement service development opportunities;
- to develop opportunities for services not currently provided by the trust;
- to shed the weaker areas of service which were being better provided elsewhere.

The strategy for the trust had to be developed in the light of a mixture of cooperation and competition from neighbouring trusts in Bristol, and within the context of a developing purchaser's strategy meeting the heath care needs of the local population.

The general strategic direction for the services of the trust has three main themes.

(i) To provide high quality, locally based, community services for the Frenchay district of about 250 000, complemented by excellent secondary care general medical, general surgical, and mental health services.

(ii) To provide high quality subregional services in neurological, plastic, burns, head and neck, and thoracic surgery.

(iii) To provide high quality major trauma services based on (i) and (ii) above.

All the activities of the trust must be directed toward achieving these goals.

Some of the existing services provided by the trust do not fit tidily into the above three strategic themes. Most, if not all of these, enhance the general services provided and in themselves represent opportunities for development, such as health promotion, forensic, and drug abuse services. A view has had to be taken about their continuation as part of the trust's services.

To complement this general strategy the trust board and the management team needed to review:

(i)   the strategic direction for services for the next five years;
(ii)   the strengths and weaknesses of services currently provided;
(iii)   service development opportunities for the trust;
(iv)   development opportunities for services not currently provided by the trust;
(v)   prospective strategies of the purchasing authorities and fundholders.

In pursuing the strategy for service provision, a degree of uncertainty exists in defining:

(i)   the strategic direction of the main purchaser;
(ii)   the extending role and responsibility of general practice fundholders;
(iii)   the requirements of the Patient's Charter and other national directives;
(iv)   the extent to which fundholders will "buy" community staff and services;
(v)   the rate at which priorities will be pursued in *Health of the Nation* targets;
(vi)   the extent to which more distant purchasers will wish to invest in "local" contracts;
(vii)   the impact of community care legislation;
(viii) the financial resources available to purchasers;
(ix)   advances in the practice of medicine;
(x)   statutory training requirements for staff;
(xi)   changes in demography in the population;
(xii)   the balance between cooperation and competition with neighbouring trusts.

The trust has to be flexible in determining its marketing policy so that it can adapt to changing circumstances. Thus all directorates have had to identify strengths, weaknesses, threats and opportunities for their services as part of their business plans.

The organisational structure in Frenchay has proved particularly appropriate for pursuing this strategy. The clinical directors have been able to develop both the services provided by their own directorates as well as developing the strategy of the whole organisation. Even so, such a cohesive structure does not confer immunity from the problems of functioning in a market orientated environment, illustrated by the case study.

Case study

In March 1993 the trust learned for certain that its 1993–4 contract income would be £1.3m less than expected and that it would have to find a further £1.0m to meet other unavoidable costs (cost pressures). Thus income would be £2.3m less than expenditure.

The management team had been aware that there could be a small shortfall. The final "bill" for savings, however, was much higher than originally anticipated due to the late agreement of contracts. The management team agreed a set of principles to guide the process of making the necessary savings.

(i) Managerial costs and non-clinical overheads would bear the brunt of the savings.

(ii) Savings would be made in an objective and rational way. The principle that emergency admissions would always be accepted would be protected.

(iii) The savings should have a minimal impact on patient care. First priority would be given to maintaining and developing high quality patient care services.

(iv) Facilities required to provide patient services would be rationalised to match the lower contracts. This meant that the clinical directors would look at the facilities they needed to meet their contracts and that existing facilities would be slimmed down or extended, based on those needs.

(v) The need for savings and the ways of making them must be understood, accepted, and owned by the clinical directors, the consultant body, and by all managers in the organisation.

(vi) The need for the reduction in expenditure must be explained to the entire workforce. Only by maintaining excellent communications with the workforce would it be possible to keep their support through what was clearly going to be a difficult and taxing exercise. This task fell largely to the chief executive.

Clinical directors were expected, with their managers, to devise the cost savings and match the facilities required to meet contracts and then to implement the proposals, doing their utmost to keep all staff fully informed of the reasons behind this process.

All clinical directors were asked to: check the accuracy of their budgets; advise the management team on mismatch of facilities against contract; test their services against a potential 1%, 2%, and 5% cost saving target while maintaining necessary and agreed developments.

These were hard tasks and in this relatively young organisation it was the first time that the clinical directors had had to shoulder the responsibility of deciding where major reductions in expenditure could or should be made. The clinical directors themselves had learnt enough to understand the necessity for the reductions and one of the early and major tasks was for them to convince the consultants and other professional staff within their directorates.

The merits of the organisational structure began to shine through. For instance, several consultants did not take kindly to being told that their operating time or beds, or both, would have to be curtailed because of fewer contracts, but it became clear that this message was more acceptable coming from a consultant colleague than from a "manager" because the clinical director was perceived as appreciating the clinical consequences of the measures being advocated.

Where to reduce costs

Each clinical director, in conjunction with his general manager, examined the performance of the various functions within the directorate, matched this performance with the newly agreed contract volumes, and explored ideas for reductions in expenditure. In the acute bed directorates (surgery, medicine, and neurosciences) numbers of beds were compared with contract levels, projected duration of patient stay, needs for investigations, drugs, and theatre time. Emergency workloads provided one of the biggest problems as in medicine and surgery this was not subject to control. The reduced contract volumes could therefore only be matched against elective work which then became a smaller proportion of the total workload, and, therefore, made the service's ability to cope with a variable and unknown workload that much more difficult. A similar exercise was undertaken within the mental health and community directorates.

In the more service orientated directorates (clinical facilities and clinical support) services were matched against the projected reduced demand.

How to reduce costs

Tough decisions then had to be taken by the management team about the ways in which the savings would be made and the possible effects on the quality of the clinical services and the

---

Clinical directorates

Surgery:	General
	Gynaecology
	Thoracic
	Trauma and orthopaedics
	Plastic
	Oral and maxillo–facial
Neuroscience:	Neurosurgery
	Neurology
	Neuropathology
	Neurophysiology
	Neuropsychiatry
	Speech therapy
	Physiotherapy
Clinical	Radiology (including neuroradiology)
support	Pathology (excluding neuropathology)
	Pharmacy
Clinical	Accident and Emergency
facilities:	Operating theatres and endoscopy unit
	CSSD and TSSU
	Anaesthesia (including ICU and pain clinic)
	Daycase unit
	Outpatient department
	Medical physics
	Medical illustration
Mental health:	Acute psychiatry and rehabilitation
	Forensic psychiatry
	Challenging behaviour
	Drug misuse service
	Community psychiatry
	Psychiatry of old age
	Clinical psychology
Medicine:	Acute medicine
	Care of the elderly
	Occupational therapy
	Dietetics
Community:	Community paediatric services
	Child and adolescent psychiatry
	District nursing and health visiting
	Chiropody

---

support services. There was much agonising over the continuing need for investment in the various services. In the main the trust's list of "necessary developments" contained items identifying changes in clinical practice which our main purchaser did not recognise as being a priority for investment but which had already been implemented as being improvements in patient care. These included increased use of isotopes, higher costs of drugs due to an increased number of emergency admissions, implants for spinal surgery, and disposables for laparascopic surgery. Continued use of these techniques was debated at length before being authorised.

The outcome of the reviews by the clinical directors identified that about 152 staff would be at risk of redundancy and 35 staff would be downgraded. The problem was lessened by there having been a "freeze" on the filling of all vacancies as soon as the problem had been recognised. A trust steering group had been set up to which requests for the filling of vacancies were submitted. Whenever feasible, short term contracts were offered.

Due to the foresight of the management team and the hard work of the clinical directors and their managers most of the "at risk" staff had been either redeployed or re-employed in the organisation within three months. Most of the remainder had accepted early retirement or voluntary redundancy.

Role of the clinical director

The critical factor in producing a successful and workable plan was the real involvement of the clinical director in developing proposals for their own services and promoting the need for change among their clinical colleagues, and the need to be involved in the process. This was coupled with the trust which existed between the clinical directors, the chief executive, the other members of the management team, and the cadre of specialty directors.

The execution of the implementation plan for 1993–4 really tested the trust's version of the involvement of the clinicians in management. The clinical directors, without having any managerial authority over their clinical colleagues, had to manage a cost savings exercise which would affect them all. The chief executive had to resist the temptation to intervene when problems loomed— the clinical directors had to be given the opportunity to consolidate their managerial credibility. She acted as a sounding board and adviser and intervened only when it was necessary to reinforce the decisions of the clinical directors.

As a result of the exercise, the trust's expenditure was reduced in line with its income and the trust was one of the few which met all its financial targets.

The lessons

When the problem first arose it was tempting, and would have been all too easy, to adopt the conventional solution and insist that the problem be solved by the general managers rather than through the agreed structure. This, however, would have undermined the principles on which the structure had been based. Four major difficulties still remain:

- The demands on the time of the chief executive;
- The demands on the time of the clinical directors and their specialty colleagues;
- The perceived interruption of the career paths of the general managers;
- The potential tensions arising from functional directors, such as finance, delegating responsibility to clinicians and not traditional managers.

The organisation is now far better placed to undertake major projects and initiatives than it was before: decisions are multidimensional and largely consensual; managers and clinicians work in harmony together. The clinical directors are not disenfranchised but are an essential part of the decision making

---

Effectiveness of a clinical directorate

- Clinical directors have to be given real responsibility for the delivery of the clinical service of their directorate

- Such responsibility must include budgetary control, staff management, and contract management

- Clinical directors must have good quality management, nursing, financial and information support

- There must be no intervening layer of management between the chief executive and the clinical directors

- The chief executive must be able to adopt a "hands off" approach to operational management while ensuring the strategic aims of the organisation are fulfilled and that the clinical directors are fully supported in making their decisions

- This is not a cheap system of management, but the full integration of the clinicians brings benefits which far outweigh the additional costs

process in the trust. They are readily accepted by their consultant colleagues as acting in the clinical interests of patients.

We believe that the strengths of our clinical directorate model of management, with its direct access to the chief executive, lead to realistic and robust decisions which minimise disruption to the services, make for faster decision making, and maximise benefits to patient care.

There are several lessons to be learnt from the experiences outlined above as they affected Frenchay Healthcare Trust.

We believe that this system of management has allowed decisions concerning the future of the services provided and their current performance and potential to be taken by the clinical staff and managers working together to achieve a common goal. It has allowed a synergy to prosper between the aims and objectives of these two groups of staff that is changing the culture of the organisation. It has focused on the importance of decisions being taken by staff with a shared perspective, particularly in times of change.

Key point summary

- Strategic direction needs to be established early, determining what is to be provided and how this is to be achieved
- Flexibility is important: the identification of strengths and weaknesses, and threats and opportunities for the directorate needs to be part of the business plan
- A clinical directorate model of management, with direct access to the chief executive, minimises disruption to service provision, while maximising patient care
- The effectiveness of a clinical directorate depends on being given real responsibility and on good support systems

---

7 Making finance work for you — strategic issues in clinical directorates

JOHN STUART, PETER C SPURGEON, ANTHONY COOK

The NHS has a long history of underinvestment interspersed with periodic bouts of overspending to relieve the ensuing crises. Strict cash limits make it unlikely that funding will match the multiple demands of an increasingly aging population, rising drug prices, and advancing technology. In this context it is difficult to perceive the finance function as a "flexible friend."

The restructuring of the NHS, with the formation of budget holding clinical teams (directorates) and self governing (trust) status for hospitals, and especially contracting, which brings together activity and financial data, means that clinicians now have the opportunity to influence the use of revenue funds in a more imaginative way than before, to improve patient care. Yet, many doctors view financial management as yet another mechanism for restricting clinical freedom. But doctors who participate actively in financial management within a sufficiently large clinical directorate can make finance work to achieve a clinical service of more uniform quality.

To illustrate the point, we have compiled a case history which is not based on any one hospital or health authority. We begin with a clinical service directorate (surgery) and follow with a support service directorate (laboratory medicine).

64

Case study

Bottomless Memorial Hospital is a large district general hospital in an urban health authority which also contains one other general hospital and a specialist hospital for the elderly. The three hospitals have recently amalgamated to achieve self governing NHS trust status (Bottomless Trust Hospitals). There has been little or no collaboration between the hospitals in the past, but a new management structure with clinical directorates extending across all three hospitals has now been established by a new chief executive. A computerised clinical information system is also being developed as part of the NHS resource management initiative. Serious financial difficulties in both clinical and support services have yet to be resolved.

Clinical services (surgery)

The financial difficulties within Bottomless Trust Hospitals include surgery, which, for the current financial year, was funded by a contract for £3m (on an historical basis this would treat 3000 patients) that was not sensitive to workload (block contract). Six months into the financial year 1600 patients had been treated and actual expenditure was £1.7m.

The new surgical directorate was asked to rectify the situation by adjusting surgical activity to within budgetary guidelines. The availability of known costs for different patient categories or case

---

Factors contributing to the surgical overspend of £0.2m at six months

- 100 more patients than intended treated in six months—extra cost of £100 000 above anticipated income.

- Case mix did not match that predicted, with more expensive patient categories predominating to create an unanticipated cost of £81 400.

- One consultant led surgical team more expensive (£18 600 additional cost over six months) than others; this team also had a 1.5 day longer than average length of ward stay and a longer waiting list despite a similar case mix.

65

mix enabled the surgical business manager to identify several factors that had contributed to the deficit (box).[1]

The following strategy was therefore devised by the surgical directorate.

Rationalise the surgical service

The service was rationalised across the two general hospitals, with the major surgical specialties transferred to Bottomless Memorial Hospital to allow the other hospital to concentrate on general surgery and day case surgery. Costs were reduced by converting some of the inpatient beds to day beds.

Calculate accurate costs

Streaming of surgical cases across hospitals in this way facilitated the calculation of the cost per case for laboratory tests, consumables, and length of stay. The surgical business manager was thus able to plan a better mix of high, medium, and low cost cases for contracting purposes, and proposed a move towards a new (cost and volume) contract which would be sensitive to workload.

Investigate variance in performance

Investigation of the cause of the longer than average ward stay of one consultant's patients revealed overcommitted junior staff and a consultant with insufficient sessions on that site. As a result, meetings of the clinical team to plan patient discharges and maximise throughput were irregular. Costs for drugs and consumables were also disproportionately high. Surgical sessions were rescheduled to reduce the consultant's commitments on the other site, and more frequent patient review rounds were agreed. The business manager also identified that the appointment of a part time laboratory phlebotomist from 7.00-9.00 am would result in earlier blood count results and facilitate patient discharges.

The surgeons supported these proposals for rationalisation across the hospitals because they addressed their own concerns for clinical priorities, including quality of service to patients and advances in day case surgery, as well as addressing financial concerns.

Support services (laboratory medicine)

Laboratory services in the three hospitals had suffered from underinvestment, resulting in a build up of aging equipment and reliance on labour intensive work practices; staff accounted for more than 80% of costs. The chief executive had declared that a 10% savings target (recurring) was required from the revenue budget of £5m for the combined laboratories. The following financial strategy was therefore adopted by the pathologists.

Establishing the correct start budget

While £5m accurately reflected the sum of each of the laboratory budgets, the pathologists identified hidden support costs within the finance, personnel, and other management services of each hospital. It was therefore agreed to transfer a further £0.1m to the new laboratory medicine directorate. The first financial objective, of maximising the start budget by accurately identifying all components, was therefore achieved.

Rationalising the analytical service

The pathologists realised that they would have to free sufficient income not only to meet the savings target but also to raise service quality in the future. This, they realised, could be achieved by amalgamating the historically separate analytical services of the three hospitals.

The Audit Commission has stated that laboratory savings can best be achieved by centralising the staff and equipment required for specialist tests.[2] As an acute laboratory service on the two district general hospital sites was an agreed quality requirement, there was no plan to centralise all diagnostic services to one hospital. It was therefore agreed to centralise to Bottomless Memorial Hospital those specialist and routine tests that did not require a result within four hours. A motor cycle courier service was contracted to provide a rapid transport link. To process the remaining work on the other district general hospital site the previously separate pathology disciplines were amalgamated into a single multidisciplinary laboratory which was relocated next to the outpatient–casualty areas and linked by a dedicated pneumatic tube delivery system to the intensive care unit. This improved the turnround time of the results service, produced revenue savings, and eliminated the cost of additional instruments for near patient testing. The small laboratory at the hospital for the elderly was closed and the service thereafter provided from the central laboratory, making use of the courier service.

Improving preanalytical and postanalytical services

Laboratories often lack control over their preanalytical (blood collection, specimen transport) and postanalytical (return of test reports to clinicians) services. Both phases are critical determinants of laboratory response time, particularly when services are centralised; the completion time of test requests is becoming an increasingly important measure of quality for diagnostic laboratories. It was agreed that the laboratory medicine directorate would now hold the budget for phlebotomists and laboratory porters and drivers. This is a further example of correct identification of the start budget.

Computer systems are essential in laboratory medicine: benefits range from modification of the requesting behaviour of clinicians by the use of expert systems[3-5] to the rapid return of results. Funds from the health authority's information technology budget were therefore allocated for a standard computer system to link all laboratories on the two sites and to link the laboratories with the hospital clinical information system. These improvements to the preanalytical and postanalytical phases of laboratory testing improved service quality.

Introduction of zero based, flexible budgeting

Support services need financial protection from unplanned and unfunded increases in demand by clinicians. This can be achieved for selected services by a combination of zero based and flexible budgeting. This entails a move from a fixed budget, allocated according to historical levels of demand, to a budget that can change according to the level of clinical activity but which starts at zero. The required income is then recovered from each clinical directorate in proportion to use of the service. The blood and blood products budget and the on call service were therefore selected for zero based, flexible budgeting because the pathologists anticipated that they would have little control over demand; the budget holding clinical directorates, on the other hand, could audit their own use of these services.

Leasing rather than buying equipment

In the above case study there had been no capital investment to replace the aging equipment and thereby increase efficiency through automation. The alternative was to lease equipment.

Capital equipment funds have been eroded so frequently in the NHS that the leasing of equipment is becoming the favoured option in many instances. The pathologists found that the financial terms offered by instrument manufacturers were highly negotiable and favoured lease over purchase as capital charges were required to be paid on any equipment purchased by the directorate.[6] Lease of equipment also included an attractive price for consumables. Thus the intrinsically higher costs of leasing were largely offset within the financial package, as well as by future revenue savings arising from automation.

Thus, by imaginative restructuring, the laboratory directorate created new financial opportunities. Investment in the laboratory service was provided by the chief executive for information technology and for refurbishing the laboratories, in view of the clear financial and quality benefits of the strategic plan. As staff costs still consumed more than 80% of revenue costs in the main laboratory a reduction in staff numbers by cross discipline working patterns and an alteration in skills mix was planned. This would generate further savings, facilitate a move towards a 24 hour laboratory service (replacing on call), and justify the cost of a pneumatic tube system to replace in part the portering service. Market testing of the laboratory service was not imposed by the chief executive as it would not have been timely to introduce this further variable during the agreed restructuring process.

Conclusion

The strategies outlined in this case study incorporate several general principles that allowed finance to be used more effectively. The principal gain arose from the opportunity to rationalise services between previously separate hospitals and clinical teams. Such opportunities are now possible as a consequence of the restructuring of the NHS and should be used to correct the erosion of quality which often occurs when an inadequate budget is spread over too many cost centres. Unfortunately the formation of multiple self governing trusts within some health authorities limits such rationalisation and as yet there is little experience of collaboration between trusts. Rationalisation does require team work, as opposed to the freedom of independent clinical units, but working as a team within a large directorate can achieve the critical mass required to maintain, and make more uniform, the quality of the service.

The strategy behind making finance work for you at clinical directorate level is not complex, the more detailed aspects of budget management being the responsibility of the directorate's business manager. What is more demanding at clinical director level is the management skill required to implement change and achieve a synergy between the directorate and hospital management to ensure purposeful implementation of agreed strategy.

1 Perrin J. *Resource management in the NHS*. Wokingham: Van Nostrand Reinhold, 1988: 86–141.
2 Audit Commission for Local Authorities and the National Health Service in England and Wales. *The pathology services: a management review*. London: HMSO, 1991.
3 Gama R, Nightingale PG, Broughton PMG, Peters M, Ratcliffe JG, Bradby GVH, *et al*. Modifying the requesting behaviour of clinicians. *J Clin Pathol* 1992: **45**: 248–9.
4 Mutimer D, McCauley B, Nightingale P, Ryan M, Peters M, Neuberger J. Computerised protocols for laboratory investigation and their effect on use of medical time and resources. *J Clin Pathol* 1992; **45**: 572–4.
5 Peters M, Broughton PMG. The role of expert systems in improving the test requesting patterns of clinicians. *Ann Clin Biochem* 1993; **30**: 52–9.
6 Cook AN. The NHS reforms and the finance functions. In: Spurgeon P, ed. *The new face of the NHS*. Harlow: Longman, 1993: 46–71.

Key point summary

- Services can be rationalised (amalgamated) to address financial concerns, while still maintaining and even improving quality of service

- A start budget needs to be accurate: identify all component costs, including hidden support costs

- Centralise or rationalise staff and equipment for specialist tests

- To increase efficiency, computerise where possible, and consider lease rather than purchase of equipment

- Introduce zero based, flexible budgeting for selected services instead of a fixed budget allocated on the basis of previous demand

- Reduce staff costs, often one of the largest overheads, by cross discipline working patterns and a change in the skills mix of staff

8 Financial accounting in the NHS

ANTHONY COOK

Just as the NHS is changing, so is the world of finance and financial management within it. Indeed, although recent changes appear to be particularly far reaching, the process of change has been with us since at least the NHS reorganisation in 1974.

To understand recent changes in financial management within the NHS one should first of all understand the distinction between *financial* accounting and *management* accounting.

Financial accounting

Financial accounting (also sometimes known as *stewardship* accounting) is the process whereby any organisation needs to have systems in place simply to enable transactions to take place. Wages and salaries have to be paid, supplies (such as drugs) or services (such as electricity) have to be bought, and income has to be collected from customers. All of these transactions have to be conducted properly. In the case of paying salaries for example, this means not only paying the right salary to the right employee at the right time but also making the right deductions for income tax, national insurance, and pensions contributions; remitting *that* money to the appropriate authorities; and maintaining the necessary records. In due course these records are summarised to produce (usually) annual accounts. Only in a few comparatively minor respects are the principles of financial accounting any different in the NHS from any other large organisation.

Historically, modern financial accounting grew out of the industrial revolution of the nineteenth century. Large scale industrial enterprises could be created only with substantial inputs of capital. This in turn required that investors needed to be found and persuaded to part with their money. They in their turn expected a return on their investment and also *an account* of how the organisation had fared over the previous year. The format of modern financial accounts has therefore grown from the separation of *the ownership* of an organisation (the investors or shareholders) from the enterpreneurial *management* of the organisation. The financial accounts represent the "accounts" that the managers are required to give to the owners of how their resources have been deployed.

Entity Concept

Management accounting

Management accounting, in contrast, is concerned with producing financial information to help the management of the organisation. This information can be required for decision making, for producing financial or business plans, or for facilitating financial control. Management accounting is different in nature from financial accounting and the key differences are summarised in the box.

The question is not whether management accounting is better or more important than financial accounting, or vice versa. Rather, every organisation must have its financial accounting—perhaps as its basic building blocks—but its management

---

Differences between financial and management accounts

	Financial accounts	Management accounts
Accounts to:	The owners of the organisation	The management of the organisation
Produced:	Annually	Frequently
Detail:	Summary	May be highly detailed
Format:	Specified	Left to local discretion
Time perspective:	Historical	Forward looking

accounting will grow out of its financial accounting. In large organisations both are essential.

Before the *Working for Patients* white paper the changes which occurred in the NHS during the 1970s and 1980s were primarily concerned with the development of management accounting. Following the creation of the internal market the changes are impacting on financial accounting in the NHS. In due course the pendulum will swing back towards management accounting.

For the time being, however, the emphasis is on developments affecting financial accounting, and nowhere are the changes more in evidence than in the accounting regime of NHS trusts.

Accounting within trusts

NHS trusts, of course, are an integral part of the newly reorganised NHS. In the internal market of purchasers and providers they are providers: hospital and community units given a legal status in their own right, independent of the managerial control of their local district health authority, and competing with other providers to secure business from their local purchasers. They are being pitched into a deliberately commercial environment, and they must behave in a commercial way. The accounting regime is similarly commercial and displays many of the features of the accounts of private sector limited companies.

Double entry book keeping

Let us begin at the beginning with *double entry book keeping*. Its principles are commonly attributed to an Italian merchant, Paciolo, in the fifteenth century. He realised that there are two sides to every transaction and therefore there should be two entries in the books of accounts to record it. Thus, if I go into my local newsagents to buy a magazine, on the one hand I come out clutching my copy of *Management Today*; on the other hand, I have parted with my money. If I am recording the transaction in my own books of account I have purchased the magazine (the debit entry) and I have reduced my holding of cash (the credit entry). Every transaction in every organisation involves two entries—the debits and the credits. And at the end of each accounting period the first test of the accuracy of the entries is to see that all the debits add up to the same total as all the credits. This is the *trial balance*.

Once the trial balance is completed we can move on to the end of year accounts. Double entry books in fact give two end of year accounts. Firstly, there is what is known in a commercial undertaking as the *profit and loss account* or in a not for profit organisation the *income and expenditure account*. Secondly, there is the *balance sheet*.

Income and expenditure account and balance sheet

The income and expenditure account, as its name implies, summarises the income received and the expenditure incurred over a period. Hence, it will usually read "Income and expenditure account *for the year ended* 31 March 19XX." In any organisation the income and expenditure account will look something like that shown in the box.

In contrast the *balance sheet* shows the situation at a particular moment—technically probably midnight on the last day of the financial year. Hence it is usually headed "Balance sheet *as at 31 March 19XX*." There are two sides to the balance sheet—which by definition, balance. Traditionally, they used to be shown side by side but nowadays are usually in the "narrative" format showing the capital employed in the business and how that capital has been funded.

Within the capital employed there will be sections for the *fixed assets*: the value of land, buildings, equipment, and motor vehicles owned by the organisation. The *current assets* will show the value of *stocks* of finished goods, work in progress, and raw materials;

Typical income and expenditure account

Income and expenditure account for the year ended 31 March 1994

INCOME	£000s	£000s
Contract income		12 137
LESS EXPENDITURE		
Materials	4109	
Wages and salaries	4983	
Services	1794	
Depreciation	1025	
	———	11 911
SURPLUS FOR YEAR		226

debtors—the money owed to the organisation by its customers; and *cash and bank accounts*. The *current liabilities* include its *creditors* (the money the organisation owes to its suppliers) and *bank overdrafts* and other *short term loans*. The current assets less the current liabilities give the total of the *working capital*—that capital which every business must have but which is necessarily tied up in reusable or recirculating assets. Then the total of the fixed assets, plus working capital, gives the total capital employed in the organisation.

That total is balanced by the sources of funding. There can be three sources of funding: (a) capital invested by the shareholders of the organisation (*share capital*); (b) any long term borrowings of the organisation (usually in the form of *debentures*, which are loans

Balance sheet as at 31 March 1994

CAPITAL EMPLOYED	£000s	£000s
Fixed assets		
Land and buildings		5936
Equipment and vehicles		6473
		12 409
Current assets		
Debtors	1759	
Stocks	2107	
Cash at bank	524	
	4390	
Less current liabilities		
Creditors	1034	
Working capital	——	3356
TOTAL CAPITAL EMPLOYED		15 765
REPRESENTED BY		
Issued share capital		8000
Plus accumulated reserves		3765
		11 765
Long term loans and debentures		4000
		15 765

secured on the assets); and (c) the accumulated retained surpluses or losses from the operations of the organisation (*accumulated reserves*).

The balance sheet in our hypothetical organisation may look something like that in the box.

At two points there are specific links between the income and expenditure account and the balance sheet. The first is the figure for "accumulated reserves" in the balance sheet. This is where the surplus from the income and expenditure account will be added (or deducted if there is a loss) and is the reason why the balance sheet always balances. Hence, our example income and expenditure account shows that a surplus of £226 000 was earned last year. In the balance sheet this might mean that there is an extra £226 000 cash in the bank. More probably, however, it is tied up in the form of additional fixed assets or stocks of raw materials and work in progress. Wherever it is, the capital employed has been enhanced by that £226 000. However, the balance sheet *does* balance because the accumulated reserves figure has also increased by £226 000 from £3 539 000 in the previous year's balance sheet to £3 765 000.

The second point at which there is a specific and obvious link between the balance sheet and the income and expenditure account is in respect of accounting for fixed assets. The value of the organisation's fixed assets is shown on the balance sheet. However, fixed assets wear out and this wear and tear is shown on the income and expenditure accounts as *depreciation*. There are several variants of accounting for fixed assets and depreciation, but the most straightforward is the *straight line* method of depreciation on *historical cost* basis. Let us assume, for example, that the organisation buys a piece of equipment for £10 000 on 31 March year 1. In the balance sheet drawn up at midnight on that date that item will appear as £10 000. Let us also assume that the item is expected to have a working life of 10 years. On the straight line method, therefore, there will be an annual depreciation figure of £1000. Thus, the depreciation figure in the income and expenditure account for year 2 will include £1000 for this item and it will appear in the balance sheet at 31 March year 2 at a written down value of £9000. Similarly, the income and expenditure account for year 3 will include £1000 depreciation on this item and the balance sheet at 31 March year 3 will include the item at a written down value of £8000.

Accruals accounting versus cash flow accounting

Thus, we have our two basic statements of account produced from our double entry book keeping: the income and expenditure account and the balance sheet. Normally these will have been prepared in accord with what accountants refer to as the *accruals concept* of accounting. Under the accruals concept an organisation will endeavour to relate income to the accounting period in which it has actually been earned—that is, when it has accrued—and expenditure to the accounting period in which resources have actually been consumed. This, of course, is different from when the payments from customers are actually received or when bills are actually paid. If we are thinking in these terms we are thinking in *cash* terms.

To illustrate the differences let us look at one or two examples. On the income side if an organisation receives a deposit on 31 March year 1 for work to be done during the next financial year, then—accounting on an *accruals* basis—that will appear on the balance sheet at 31 March under current liabilities—in effect as work owing at that moment to its customers. Accounting on a *cash basis*, of course, would appear as cash received in year 1. Alternatively, work might be completed during year 1, but payment may not be received from the customers until year 2. On an *accruals* basis of accounting the income and expenditure accounts for year 1 will show that as income earned and the balance sheet at 31 March year 1 will include that income within the organisation's debtors. When accounting on a *cash* basis the item does not appear until year 2.

We have the same effects on the expenditure side. A batch of raw materials bought and paid for but not consumed before 31 March year 1 will on, an *accruals* basis, not appear as expenditure during year 1 but will be included in the value of stocks in the balance sheet at that date. On a *cash* basis it does appear as year 1 expenditure. In contrast, electricity consumed by an organisation during March should appear on an *accruals* basis as March expenditure (and in the 31 March balance sheet as a current liability), even though it will not be paid for until the next financial year—when of course, it would appear on a *cash* basis.

While accountants will vehemently argue for the accruals basis, the director of finance must nevertheless monitor the cash position. The world of commerce abounds with examples of organisations which have gone out of business even though they are showing healthy *accruals* profits. Too much of their money has become tied up in new plant and machinery or stocks of materials or is still owed to them by their debtors, and they have simply run out of cash to pay their creditors. The point at which a business actually ceases to exist is when they can no longer pay their bills. Hence the need to monitor the cash position.

Funds flow statement

This introduces the third of our end of year financial statements: the *funds flow statement* (historically known as the *source and application of funds statement*). This is a statement which shows where the cash has come from and where it has gone to. In its simplest form it can be reconciled to the income and

---

Typical funds flow statement—when cash flow is healthy

Funds flow statement at 31 March 1994

	£000s	£000s
Operating surplus		226
Plus depreciation		1025
		1251
Movements in working capital		
Increase in debtors	207	
Increase in stocks	321	
	528	
Less increase in creditors	157	
		371
		880
Less capital expenditure		1550
		−670
Plus increase in long term loans		750
NET INCREASE IN CASH		80

---

expenditure account and the opening and closing balance sheets for the year. It might start with the operating surplus for the year and then add on the depreciation (which is not a cash item—hence if an organisation makes a £10 000 profit *after* charging £2000 depreciation the actual cash inflow is £12 000) and then show movements in working capital (increases or decreases in debtors, creditors, and stocks) together with actual capital expenditure and cash movements as further loans are taken out or repaid.

In our hypothetical organisation a relatively healthy funds flow statement for the year might look something like that in the box.

Thus while our closing balance sheet at 31 March 1994 shows cash at bank of £524 000 the opening balance sheet at 31 March 1993 would have shown a cash figure of £444 000.

If the business, however, has failed adequately to control its working capital movements and has negotiated an increase in its long term loans of only £500 000 then we would have an alternative funds flow statement.

Funds flow statement—when cash flow is inadequate

Funds flow statement at 31 March 1994

	£000s	£000s
Operating surplus		226
Plus depreciation		1025
		1251
Movement in working capital		
Increase in debtors	429	
Increase in stocks	457	
	886	
Less increase in creditors	73	
		813
		438
Less capital expenditure		1550
		−1112
Plus increase in long term loans		500
NET INCREASE IN CASH		−612

Balance sheet relating to poor funds flow statement

Balance sheet as at 31 March 1994

CAPITAL EMPLOYED	£000s	£000s
Fixed assets		
Land and buildings		5936
Equipment and vehicles		6473
		12 409
Current assets		
Debtors	1981	
Stocks	2243	
	4224	
Less current liabilities		
Creditors	1034	
Overdraft	168	
	1118	
Working capital		3106
TOTAL CAPITAL EMPLOYED		15 515
REPRESENTED BY		
Issued share capital		8000
Plus accumulated reserves		3765
		11 765
Long term loans and debentures		3750
		15 515

This in turn would give us a new closing balance sheet (notwithstanding that the business has earned the same accruals profit).

Our organisation is now in trouble. It has a bank overdraft of £168 000; it would expect to pay its creditors about £600 000 in the coming month; and it should pay wages and salaries of more than £400 000. If it diligently pursues its debtors it might pull in £1m. However, almost certainly the director of finance will need to seek additional short term finance from the bank and will probably also be looking to secure additional long term funds. Accordingly, to monitor such movements the funds flow statement is seen as an essential part of the year end accounts.

Having set out the basic principles of the year end accounting regime which apply in most large organisations, and which are specified under the Companies Acts, how, then, are these principles applied in NHS trusts? In fact, there is very little difference. NHS trusts now produce an income and expenditure account and a balance sheet (both on the *accruals* basis of accounting) and a funds flow statement. Increasingly, their annual reports and accounts are following a similar glossy format to those produced by many public limited companies.

Trusts and capital charges

What is of interest is the way they are effectively being monitored and directed by the NHS Executive. Following the publication of the *Working For Patients* white paper the initial impressions were that NHS trusts were to be dynamic, free wheeling entrepreneurial organisations vigorously competing with one another in the NHS internal market and able to develop their services in accord with their own commercial judgment.

In fact, it is now clear that NHS trusts are subject to very tight financial regulation. Before the secretary of state's revision of the "intermediate tier" the NHS Executive had established six formal outposts whose remit was to monitor the activities of NHS trusts within their zone. Each trust has to produce an annual business plan and is expected to deliver actual results in accord with that plan. To understand how this is done, we need to look at some of the details of the new NHS trust regimes.

Firstly, it is only since 1 April 1991 that the NHS has had full balance sheets. It was one of the requirements of the reforms that *asset registers* were to be created showing the value for each authority or trust of its fixed assets. In parallel with the asset registers we have had the introduction of *capital charges*—the NHS equivalent of depreciation. However, NHS practice differs from commercial practice in that the capital charges include the depreciation of fixed assets *plus* a 6% return on their capital value (this applies both within NHS trusts and directly managed units).

Secondly, if we look at the funding side of the balance sheet, we will find that it is split (in most cases originally on a 50/50 basis) between public dividend capital and interest bearing debt. These correspond to, respectively, the issued share capital of a commercial organisation (with, of course, the government being the only shareholder) and the long term loans and debentures—

also owing to the government. (In fact trusts may borrow money from other sources but only within the latitude provided by their external funding limit (see below).)

The financial duties imposed on an NHS trust are threefold: (a) to deliver 6% return on its capital employed; (b) to balance its budget; and (c) to live within its external funding limit. These duties apply, respectively, to its balance sheet, its income and expenditure account, and its funds flow statement.

Firstly, the 6% return on capital employed (taken from the balance sheet) is to be paid by the trust as interest on the interest bearing debt to the Department of Health.

Secondly, the income and expenditure account is expected to be in balance after charging capital charges—including, of course, the 6% return on capital.

The external funding limit is set each financial year, by the NHS Executive outpost in the light of the trust's proposed funds flow statement. It controls the level of capital expenditure the trust can undertake. If a trust has a zero external funding limit and its income and expenditure account is in balance—after charging depreciation—and it is not expecting any substantial movements in working capital, then it can undertake capital expenditure to the same amount as its depreciation. If it has a positive external funding limit then it can undertake more capital expenditure. Much to their horror some trusts were given negative external funding limits in the first couple of years of the regime. These were those that were deemed to have land and buildings surplus to their requirements and were expected to dispose of them.

Accordingly, it is now apparent that trusts are actually subject to very tight monitoring and direction. This is effected through controls applied to the three traditional statements of account: the balance sheet; the income and expenditure account; and the funds flow statement. In addition, there exists the potential for a further tightening of the screw in that if a trust turns out to be particularly profitable—earning over and above the 6% return on capital employed—it can be required to pay *dividends* on its public dividend capital.

The trust regime is a good illustration of how NHS accounting practice is increasingly following what has been common practice in the world of industry and commerce. It is probably the major item currently on the agenda of NHS financial management and it is, of course, an issue of financial accounting.

Key point summary

- A distinction needs to be drawn between financial accounting and management accounting

- Financial accounting is the process whereby systems need to be set up in an organisation to allow financial transactions (such as payment of salaries and purchase of services) to take place: it does not produce information to help in the management of that organisation

- The development of trusts as a result of the NHS reforms means that accounting practice is becoming more and more commercially orientated, with the emphasis, for the moment, on financial accounting

9 Management accounting

ANTHONY COOK

There is a distinction to be made between financial accounting and management accounting. Financial accounting is concerned with having sound financial systems in place to enable routine transactions—the payment of wages and salaries, the purchase of goods and services, the collection of income from customers, etc, etc—to take place, to maintain appropriate records and to produce year end accounts. Management accounting, on the other hand, is concerned with producing financial information to assist the management of the organisation.

Back in 1978, the Royal Commission noted the almost complete absence of dynamic management accounting information in the NHS,[1] so most financial developments during the 1980s were developments in management accounting. However, the government's reforms following the 1989 *Working For Patients* White Paper have initially had an enormous impact on NHS financial accounting. In particular, the creation of the NHS trusts has been important in two respects. Firstly, they need their own finance departments—with all the appropriate systems—within the trust. Previously such systems were usually located within the district health authority. This has entailed a massive reorganisation of finance departments. Secondly, trusts are subject to a three point financial regime which affects their balance sheet, their income and expenditure account, and their funds flow statement. Now that the restructuring of the NHS is nearing completion (well, maybe) the pendulum is swinging back towards management accounting.

The Chartered Institute of Management Accountants (CIMA) *Official Terminology* defines management accounting as "an integral part of management concerned with identifying, presenting and interpreting information used for:
- formulating strategy
- planning and controlling activities
- decision taking
- optimising the use of resources."[2]

Such a definition requires that we are clear about the overall objectives of the organisation. Most private sector commercial organisations might define their financial objectives as "maximising their return on capital employed," but in the public sector the financial objective must be "to deliver value for money" (VFM) from the resources provided. Furthermore, as a result of the work of the Public Accounts Committee and the National Audit Office, VFM can be expressed in terms of the three "es": economy, efficiency, and effectiveness. These terms can themselves be further defined, but for our purposes, the simplest definitions will suffice:
- economy means "doing it cheaply"
- efficiency means "doing it right"
- effectiveness means "doing the right thing"

While many would argue that effectiveness is the most important, what VFM really requires is that we must deliver effective services and we must deliver them efficiently and economically.

Perhaps the main aspect in which management accounting differs from financial accounting is the time perspective. Whereas year end (financial) accounts are historical documents, management accounting is essentially forward looking. It involves making projections, preparing plans, and asking "what happens if?"

And the type of questions to be addressed in management accounting would include:

How much does it cost to deliver our services?

How much does each activity cost?

How much does it cost to treat patients in this particular category?

Is it cheaper to contract out particular activities (such as catering, pathology, laboratories), or to provide them ourselves?

Should we build an extension to our existing hospital, or should we build a new hospital?

When should we replace our motor vehicles?

Should we replace the hospital boiler plant?

And crucially:

How can we ensure that we live within our means?

These questions can therefore be one off, requiring ad hoc investigations and reports, or they can be on going, requiring some continuous form of reporting. And it is the latter—the process of on going financial planning, monitoring, and control—which forms the core of management accounting. This process is knows as *budgetary control*.

Budgetary control, or as it is more popularly known, *budgeting* is usually an annual, cyclical process (although budgets can be prepared for longer or shorter periods). However, with a sound system of budgeting in place the other management accounting activities—whether short term ad hoc investigations, or longer term strategic plans—become much more straightforward and are built on secure foundations.

This is where budgetary systems enter the picture. A definition taken in part from an earlier (1960) management accounting terminology states: "Budgets are financial and/or quantitative statements, prepared and approved prior to a defined period of time, of the policy to be pursued during that period for the purposes of attaining given objectives."[3] Budgeting, in fact, is not just a financial exercise, but, as with management accounting in total, it is an integral part of management.

A useful starting point to understand budgeting in the NHS is the diagram (fig 9.1).[4] This shows a "three level" analysis of expenditure. Firstly, money coming into the hospital can be analysed according to what subjccts (salaries for doctors, salaries for nurses, the purchase of drugs, etc, etc) it has been spent on. Secondly, the "departmental" analysis shows "departments in which the expenditure has occurred" Thirdly, a "patient care analysis" asks on what categories of patient care has the money been spent?

The first budgets to be introduced in the NHS followed the 1974 reorganisation (which created regional health authorities and area health authorities). These were referred to as *functional* budgets. These would actually be at the second level on the diagram, but would represent budgets for each function (medical, nursing, pharmacy, etc, etc) across a hospital site, or in some cases, across an area health authority. It soon became apparent that this was actually too near the top in the managerial hierarchy

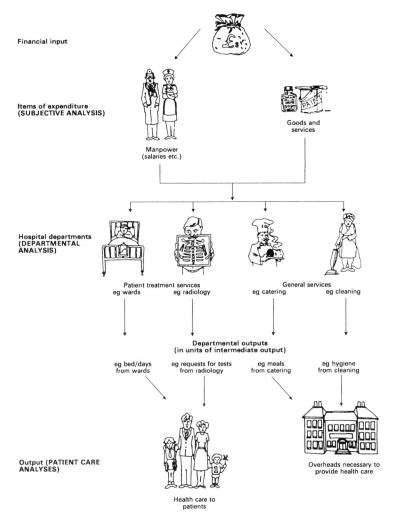

How money is used in a hospital day by day

Financial input

Items of expenditure
(SUBJECTIVE ANALYSIS)

Goods and
services

Manpower
(salaries etc.)

Hospital departments
(DEPARTMENTAL
ANALYSIS)

Patient treatment services   General services
eg wards   eg radiology   eg catering   eg cleaning

Departmental outputs
(in units of intermediate output)

eg bed/days   eg requests for tests   eg meals   eg hygiene
from wards   from radiology   from catering   from cleaning

Output (PATIENT CARE
ANALYSES)

Overheads necessary to
provide health care

Health care to
patients

Figure 9.1 Reproduced from : *The Steering Group on Health Service Information. 6th Report to the Secretary of State.* London: HMSO, 1984.

(particularly in respect of nursing) and if budgetary control was to be effective it should be devolved further down the managerial pyramid to individual departments. Hence the reference to *departmental* budgets.

According to Garbutt,[5] there are three main stages in the budgetary process:

1 *Budget setting* in which budgets are set up for agreed responsibility levels in consultation with the responsible managers.
2 *Reporting* in which the personnel for whom targets have been set are provided with information comparing actual performance with the budgets. Such compositions should lead to corrective action if necessary.
3 *Reviewing* in which budgets may be revised if business conditions change during the current period, or as a starting point for the next period.

As in any other large organisation these stages can and have been, applied in NHS acute hospitals. Table 9.1 shows a hypothetical example of a departmental budgeting statement.

Indeed if the only financial objective is the historical aim of living within the cash limit (the economy aspect of the "three es"), then many NHS hospitals have been well served by departmental budgets.

Unfortunately, that is not the end of the story. Garbutt identifies six purposes served by budgets. They are used to:

1 Allocate resources
2 Quantify plans
3 Co-ordinate departmental activities
4 Communicate management plans and objectives
5 Set performance objectives and targets
6 Plan and control business performance.

Departmental budgets certainly contribute to 1, 2, and 3, but they are seriously deficient in achieving 4, 5, and 6. That is because in a hospital fundamental objectives need to be set in clinical terms. With departmental budgets, this is not possible.

Departmental budgets are also deficient in the control aspect, because it is clinical decisions taken (predominantly) by doctors which actually incur expenditure. For example, when a doctor prescribes drugs for a patient he is actually making a financial decision, as well as a clinical one. Yet in a departmental system of budgeting the doctor is not held accountable—in financial terms—for that decision.

The corollary to that is that the departmental manager—in the NHS the chief pharmacist—is expected somehow to live within

Table 9.1 Hypothetical departmental budgeting statement

Langlands Hospital NHS Trust

Budget report: Catering Department: September 1994

	PERIOD			YEAR TO DATE		
	BUDGET £	ACTUAL £	VARIANCE £	BUDGET £	ACTUAL £	VARIANCE £
SALARIES & WAGES						
Catering manager	2000	2000		12000	12000	
Kitchen staff: Basic	18000	16800	−1200	108000	103157	−4843
Overtime		975	975		3063	3063
Canteen staff: Basic	5750	6250	500	34500	37134	2634
Overtime		155	155		907	907
SUBTOTAL	25750	26180	430	154500	156261	1761
OTHER EXPENDITURE						
Provisions	60000	70497	10497	360000	395541	35541
Other supplies	5500	4936	−564	33000	28432	−4568
Services	7500	7705	205	45000	47156	2156
SUBTOTAL	73000	83138	10138	438000	471129	33129
INCOME	−30000	−25575	4425	−180000	−155676	24324
NET EXPENDITURE	68750	83743	14993	412500	471714	59214
STAFF STATISTICS						
Catering manager	1	1		1	1	
Kitchen staff	30	28	−2	30	29	−1
Canteen staff	10	11	1	10	11	1
TOTAL STAFF	41	40	−1	41	41	
MEALS SUPPLIED						
Patients	45000	47770	2770	270000	293317	23317
Staff	15000	13532	−1468	90000	79834	−10166
TOTAL	60000	61302	1302	360000	373151	13151

his departmental budget, although he has no control over what drugs he is required to dispense and in what quantities.

Hence something better than the departmental system of budgeting is required. This is achieved in the figure by moving down from level 2 (the departmental analysis of expenditure) to level 3 (described in the diagram as "the patient care analysis," but often referred to as the *clinical* analysis of expenditure).

Just as there are differing degrees of detail, when thinking in terms of the subjective or departmental analysis of expenditure, so there are greater or lesser degrees of detail for the clinical analysis. Conventional wisdom has it that clinical expenditure can be analysed to five levels[4]:

1 *Broad client group* where one is talking in terms of "mental illness", "mental handicap," or "maternity," etc, etc.
2 *Clinical specialty* orthopaedics, paediatrics, general surgery, etc, etc.
3 *Consultant* to the clinical team of consultant and junior doctors.
4 *Disease category* in which all patients with similar complaints, and due to be treated in a similar way, are grouped together.
5 *Individual patient* How much has it cost to treat Mr Jones or Mrs Smith?

In fact, since the Royal Commission report of 1978 there have been separate initiatives concerned with analysing expenditure to each of the levels above.

In fact, analysis to client group goes back to the early 1970s and is referred to (misleadingly) as *programme budgeting*. The technique includes making broad brush assumptions about how costs can be allocated to each client group. There is nothing precise about the technique and the figures are of limited use as management information because they contain no information as to whether the resources have been used efficiently or effectively. Accordingly, programme budget figures are perhaps of greater use at the public accountability level in giving an explanation to outsiders of the way NHS resources are displayed. Recent Department of Health reports have contained "pie chart" programme budget figures.

At the next level is *specialty costing*. Specialty costs are, by definition, calculations of historical average costs per case within each specialty. Usually they are produced at the end of each financial year, although they can be (and in some cases are) produced more frequently. The technique has been in existence for some years and health authorities (and now trusts) have been required to produce specialty cost returns since the 1987/88 financial year (table 9.2). Used properly, specialty costing information can be useful for monitoring and questioning on a retrospective basis, or even planning and pricing on a prospective basis.

There have been several initiatives aimed at developing *patient costing*, which, of course, aims to calculate how much it has cost to treat each patient. Some early examples of patient costing were known as *The Financial Information Project*. Now, of course, patient costs are required in the internal market for pricing extra contractual referrals (ECRs). However, for management accounting purposes, while costs can be analysed retrospectively to the individual patient, it is not possible to plan prospectively at this level. It is not possible to predict that Mr Jones will have a heart attack next October.

Thus these three techniques—programme budgeting, specialty costing, and patient costing—are certainly of value but do not overcome all the limitations of departmental budgets. Consequently, the real need in NHS management accounting is to develop systems of *clinical budgeting*.

There were two notable early initiatives designed to concentrate at level 3—the consultant—on the clinical axis. The first of these was CASPE, which stands for Clinical and Service Planning Evaluation, and which was actually a small research group based at the King's Fund, London. CASPE dated from 1979 and the early trials concentrated on the *planning* rather than the *control* aspects of clinical budgets. Hence discussions were held with consultants and agreements drawn up as to what would be the anticiapted workload for the clinical team and what resources they would reasonably require to deliver that workload.

In 1983 the Griffiths report was published and *management budgeting* demonstration districts were established. A supporting paper written by J Blyth (unpublished) argued that the objective was:

> "to develop management budgets involving clinicians at unit level with the emphasis on management rather than accounting. The aim is to produce an unsophisticated system in which workload related budgets, covering financial and manpower allocations and full overhead costs, are closely related to workable service objectives against which performance and progress can be compared."

91

Table 9.2 Speciality and programme cost return for Walsall Hospitals NHS Trust

Patient group	Main code	Sub code	Specialties	Patients using a bed (including day cases)					Outpatients (including nurse clinic and ward attenders)			
				Patient days 56	Consultant GP episodes 57	Expenditure 58 £	Cost per patient day 59 £	Cost per episode 60 £	First attendances 61	Total attendances 62	Expenditure 63 £	Cost per attendance 64 £
B Surgical specialties												
a General surgery	200			23194	6363	5216740	224.92	819.86	4252	13466	293834	21.82
b Urology	201			8231	2596	1998665	242.82	769.90	2011	5923	188694	31.86
c Orthopaedics	202			19289	2203	3350243	173.69	1520.76	3236	13092	577244	44.09
d ENT	203			4926	2684	1434346	291.18	651.09	5021	11819	504819	42.71
e Ophthalmology	204								2303	8981	318817	35.50
f Gynaecology	205			10353	5493	2312356	223.35	420.96	2832	8952	276345	30.87
g Dental specialties	206			618	519	274080	443.50	528.09	1901	7158	409678	57.23
h Neurosurgery	207											
i Plastic surgery	208											
j Cardiothoracic	209											
k Paediatric surgery	210								39	176	8082	45.92
Subtotal B	299			66611	19858	14586430	218.98	734.54	21595	69567	2577513	37.05
C Maternity function												
a Obstetrics	301			16291	5093	3440795	211.21	675.59	4120	16051	668995	41.68
b General practice	302			1271	872	114682	90.23	131.52				
Subtotal C	399			17562	5965	3555477	202.45	596.06	4120	16051	668995	41.68
D Psychiatric specialties												
a Mental handicap	401											
b Mental illness	402											
c Child and adolescent psychiatry	403								13	91	18390	202.09
d Forensic psychiatry	404											
e Psychotherapy	405											
f Old age psychiatry	406											
Subtotal D	499								13	91	18390	202.09

This is the key paragraph in a paper which logically argued the case for clinical budgets and established a number of basic principles. Generally those principles were soundly based, although one could argue against "full overhead costs," which do not follow what is generally regarded to be good industrial or commercial practice. Similarly, the paragraph gives a clue as to why management budgeting was officially deemed to have been a failure, in that it makes reference to an "unsophisticated system." The reality is that the development of clinical budgeting systems the world over has been anything but unsophisticated.

Table 9.3 shows how management budgeting overcame several of the technical problems in developing clinical budgets. But it identified several others. It identified the need to have better information systems, particularly in respect of patient adminis-tration, radiography, pharmacy and pathology. It also identified a number of organisational and behavioural issues, in particular, what are the correct managerial relationships between the medical, nursing, and paramedical professions? To what extent can clinicians be persuaded to accept that they are financially and managerially accountable for these decisions? And does this lead to a revision of the arrangements for incorporating clinicians into the managerial structure of the hospital? It was these issues which were deemed to have been inadequately addressed in the management budgeting initiatives.

Consequently, in 1986 "management budgeting" became *resource management*, in which greater attention was to be paid to the information systems and the organisational issues. However, from a management accounting point of view, the most important change to stem from resource management was the introduction of *case mix planning and costing*. Such an approach requires that patients with similar diseases and requiring similar treatment regimens should be grouped together. It is then possible to account for the complexity of cases handled rather than the simple numbers of patients treated. In the clinical analysis of expenditure this means moving down from level 3—consultant—to level 4—disease category. The development of case mix costing is perhaps the key area in the development of health care management accounting.

The accounting objective is to establish definable categories of patients, each of which can have defined treatment regimens, and

Table 9.3 Management budgeting

Budget variance report for surgical team

	Current month			Expense codes		Year to date		
	Budget	Actual	Variance			Budget	Actual	Variance
				Staff costs controlled by team				
	10998	10697	−301	800 Medical staff costs		54990	53166	−1024
				Other expenses controlled by team				
	12499	12014	−485	809 Prescribed drugs		62495	58712	−3783
	290	248	−42	811 Histopathology – consumables		1450	1193	−257
	7697	9016	1319	820 Radiology – consumables		40837	44808	3971
	7283	7892	609	821 Operating theatre consumables		37415	38878	2463
	38767	39867	1100	Total costs controlled by team		197187	196757	570
				Costs influenced by team				
	4166	5152	986	840 Ward – consumables		20830	22584	1754
	83	149	66	841 Outpatient – consumables		415	495	80
	11572	10983	−589	845 Ward – overheads		57860	58592	732
	41	193	152	856 Outpatient – overheads		205	452	247
	1565	1782	217	849 Pharmacy – overheads		7825	8571	746
	833	814	−19	851 Histopathology – overheads		4165	4046	−119
	8208	7932	−276	861 Operating theatre – overheads		41040	40643	−397
	4107	4182	75	868 ECG – overheads		20535	21916	1381
	15485	15654	169	880 Physiotherapy–hydrotherapy		77425	75296	−2129
	46060	46841	781	Total costs influenced by team		230300	232595	2295

Table 9.3 Continued

Budget variance report for surgical team

	Current month	Code	Expense codes	Year to date	
			General services overheads		
2261	−238	890	Unit administration	11236	−1259
1028	55	891	Catering	5386	521
817	−402	892	Domestic	3932	−2163
946	114	894	Linen/laundry	4701	541
6753	−746	896	Estate management	35388	−2107
13022	−1217		Total general service overheads	65110	−4467
97849	664		Total costs for team	489995	−1602
			Memorandum statistics		
857	21	900	Inpatients – days	4382	97
148	45	903	Outpatients – attendances	740	109
499	−203	914	Histopathology – tests	2495	155
473	209	937	Radiology – tests	2801	889
599	35	940	Operating theatre – hours	2995	291

Preliminary draft for a report, with simulated cost figures, reproduced from the CASPE Project at Lewisham and North Southwark Health Authority, by permission.
Taken from *Public Sector Accounting and Financial Control.* 2nd Edition. Wokingham: Van Nostrand Reinhold.

then to build up defined treatment costs. Such an exercise involves setting standard costs for units of hospital activity, such as "occupied bed/days" or operating theatre hours, and then applying them to standard care profiles to produce—in management accounting terms, *standard product costs*. Most industrial or commercial concerns have standard costs for their product ranges, and would regard them as essential information for financial planning, budgetary control, and pricing.

The difficulties arise, of course, from the fact that, in the NHS we are dealing with patients in a hospital rather than products in a factory. Inevitably, therefore, even within the same category, some patients are more severely ill than others, some have more complications, some respond to treatment better than others, etc, etc. The real problem, therefore, with case mix costing is to identify groupings which make both medical sense—in that all patients in the group are clinically similar—and accounting sense—in that the treatment of each patient will require similar—and predictable—resources. The internal market creates a further requirement that case mix categories must make sense to purchasers—whether district health authorities or GP fundholders.

Thus the real issue is not the technicalities of the management accounting and information systems, but how to define the categories of patients. There have been several approaches to this.

For example, in the days of management budgeting Southmead developed early case mix costs for a small number of consultants. They were asked to identify the 10 or 12 case types which make up 80% or so of their routine workload. The defined treatment profile was then costed using standard costs. This approach is perfectly logical on a local basis, but it makes comparisons between sites difficult.

The most well known system is that developed at Yale University in the United States, and based on the International Disease Classification, whereby all acute patients can be allocated to one of 475 diagnosis related groups (DRGs). The Medicare system in the USA is actually funding hospitals on the basis of a price per DRG. In the United Kingdom the six original resource management sites initially started work with DRGs. However, more recently they have developed a system more suited to British practice and known as HRGs (health care resource groups). Table

Table 9.4 Hypothetical example of classification according to health care resource graphs, based on British experience

SPECIALTY : ORTHOPAEDICS

PROCEDURE : ARTHROPLASTY OF HIP

AVERAGE LENGTH OF STAY : 15 DAYS

THEATRE TIME : 1.83 HOURS

ESTIMATED COST PER CASE

	UNITS	COST PER UNIT £	COST PER CASE £
Pre-operative nursing	1.00	36.77	36.77
X-ray tests	4.20	12.78	53.67
Path Lab tests	6.50	11.75	76.37
Theatre costs	1.83	350.00	640.50
Blood	2.46	51.00	125.46
Prosthesis	1.00	545.00	545.00
Drugs	15.00	13.88	208.20
Nursing	15.00	37.00	555.00
Other L.O.S. costs	15.00	55.00	825.00
Physiotherapy	9.50	15.00	142.50
TOTAL COST			3208.47

9.4 shows a hypothetical example based on recent British experience.

Another American approach stems from the Johns Hopkins University. This recognises that even within the same disease category, some patients are more seriously ill than others and require more extensive (and more expensive) treatment. This approach has therefore introduced severity ratings to enable patients to be classified into one of four categories of severity.

The reality is that case mix costing is still in its infancy and a precise system of classification has still to be developed. However, there is no reason to assume that the problems of classification will not eventually be overcome. But it will probably require more categories coupled with severity ratings. And this overall structure for the development of clinical budgeting with case mix costing was established well before the government embarked on the NHS reforms.

Now we have the *Costing for Contracting* (CFC) initiative.[6] This is guidance stemming from the NHS Executive to acute units on how they should classify costs and allocate or apportion overhead departments, etc, specifically for the purpose of calculating prices for the internal market.[6] In fact, this addresses only one aspect and a comprehensive budgeting system can (and should) be used for planning, monitoring and control purposes, in addition to pricing. Nevertheless, CFC does follow the overall structure outlined above and it should be noted that, for the 1995/96 contracting round, trusts are required to price one of three specialties (orthopaedics, opthalmology, or gynaecology) down to HRG level. It will be interesting to see how many achieve that.

Undoubtedly, budgetary control is the core of management accounting in the NHS, just as it is in other large organisations. It provides the basis of short term financial control, ad hoc investigations, and strategic planning over a longer term period. However, when drawing up plans for a three, five, or 10 year perspective then there is a further management accounting technique that is equally important: *capital expenditure investment appraisal.* In financial accounting terms capital expenditure can be seen as expenditure of new fixed assets— land, buildings, equipment, etc. In *economic* terms, however, it can be seen as major items of expenditure incurred now, with a view to obtaining specific benefits in the future—maybe several years in the future. The investment appraisal task, therefore, is to assess whether the anticipated benefits outweigh the cost being incurred now. There are two key aspects to this process in the NHS.

Firstly, it has to be recognised that the benefits (and to some extent the costs) are incurred at different times in the future. This means that they have different values to us now. Thus the promise of a payment of £1000 in a year's time is worth considerably more to us than the promise of £1000 in 10 years' time. The approach, therefore, is to assess the *present value* of benefits and costs which can be seen as projecting forward into the future (up to 60 years in the future in the case of NHS building schemes). This involves a financial technique known as *discounting* which basically involves using compound interest in reverse. The technique in the NHS is simply a variant of the technique known as discounted cash flow (DCFs) and which is widely used by management accountants in industry and commerce.

The second aspect of investment appraisal in the NHS,

however, is that it is not possible to put a financial price on benefits achieved from better health care. It is not really possible to put a price on providing better care for the elderly, or the mentally handicapped, or even for achieving better acute care. This is in contrast to the normal commercial world where a company can usually assess in financial terms (say, additional sales of a new product) the benefits anticipated from a capital expenditure scheme. Accordingly in the NHS, there is a developing process known as the *appraisal of options*. Under this approach the basic *service need*—say, to improve maternity services in a district—is identified in the strategic planning process. Once identified, the project team must then identify a number of alternative ways in which that service need can be met. These options could involve extending an existing hospital site, building a new hospital, or even improving community services (not all of the options have to be *capital* options). It then becomes possible to assess the financial costs of each option and the non-financial benefits and then to select the preferred option.

This technique was first introduced in 1981 and was updated in 1986. It has now been further updated to take into account the complexities of the internal market with the (long awaited) release of the new *Capital Investment Manual*.[7]

Investment appraisal is, of course, a fundamental management accounting technique and enables such questions to be addressed as "Should we build a new ward for the care of the elderly?" "Should we install a new boiler plant?" or "Should we purchase the latest piece of diagnostic equipment?" It also allows us to assess the likely changes in the NHS over a strategic planning period. As with budgetary capital, it is still evolving in the context of the NHS.

In many ways the impact of the NHS reforms has been to put the development of management accounting on hold. A clear agenda existed at the end of 1988. But the overall objective must be the development of a comprehensive management accounting structure which enables NHS managers to obtain the greatest value for money from their limited resources. The process is akin to completing a jigsaw puzzle. Undoubtedly the two new developments—the *costing for contracting* guidance and the *Capital Investment Manual*—are important pieces in the jigsaw. However, many pieces are still missing.

Key point summary

- Management accounting is concerned with producing financial information to assist the management of the organisation

- Management accounting is essentially forward looking

- On going financial planning, monitoring, and budgetary control form its core

- It can be applied to the NHS so that managers can obtain the greatest value for money from their limited resources

- It is still developing in the context of the NHS

1 Royal Commission on the NHS. Research Paper No 2. *Management of financial resources in the NHS.* London: HMSO, 1978
2 Chartered Institute of Management Accountants. *Management accountancy—official terminology.* London: CIMA, 1991.
3 Institute of Cost and Works Accountants. *Terminology of cost accounting.* London: 1960.
4 DHSS. *Steering Group on Health Services Information (Chairman : Mrs E Korner) 6th Report to the Secretary of State.* London: HMSO, 1984.
5 Garbutt D. *Making budgets work.* London: Chartered Institute of Management Accountants, 1992.
6 NHS Executive. *Costing for contracting manual.* Leeds: DoH, 1993.
7 NHS Executive. *Capital investment manual.* London: HMSO, 1994.

10 Getting the best from people

ANDREW VALLANCE OWEN

Case study

A surgeon was appointed to a new consultant post in a hospital in the south of England. The advertisement for the post had given little detail and the job description was equally vague, but he had understood, through discussion before his appointment, that he would be able to develop his special interest while in the job.

On taking up the post he found out almost immediately that he had been allocated only one operating list a week when his predecessor had had three. Although he thought he had been appointed to develop a specialist role, little interest was shown in this and, despite his limited access to theatre, criticism began to be made about his developing waiting list. He soon realised that some of his consultant colleagues had been against the establishment of a new post from the start.

The situation slowly deteriorated over the next two years, although during this time he was able to build up a reasonable private practice. In his NHS hospital, he felt that staff were somehow being turned against him, including the nursing staff in theatre who had been asked to report on his attendance and punctuality, although they had never complained about this. He became increasingly concerned and frustrated over the lack of resources being put into his unit and eventually spoke out on this issue at a public meeting.

Shortly after this he was called in to account to the chief executive and medical director without being given the opportunity to bring a supporting friend. Only at the meeting itself was he given statements that had been written about him—two of them specifically commissioned—containing a number of minor allegations. He was given little chance to defend himself and threatened with the possibility of dismissal if he did not "improve."

At this point he involved the BMA which sought a meeting with personnel. When this eventually took place the personnel director opened up the completely new possibility of redundancy because of financial cutbacks; she denied that there were any formal or disciplinary charges being made against him. The whole thing had been handled so badly that it was clear he would be able to fight off this threat, but he had, by now, become so demoralised that he decided to resign his post in any case and left the NHS to work in Saudi Arabia.

In the 1950s McGregor described two very different sets of assumptions which he called Theory 'X' and Theory 'Y'.[1] Theory 'X' assumes that people are naturally lazy, lacking in ambition, and self centred, and that they need to be managed by coercion and control. Theory 'Y' assumes that people are not naturally like this, but if they become so it is due to their experiences, that they are ready to assume responsibility and getting the best out of them needs management which is collaborative and supportive. Theory 'Y' is the philosophy on which this article is based.

Although details have been changed to preserve anonymity, the case study is based on an amalgam of real experiences in this country over the past two years. It shows effectively how to demotivate comprehensively a young consultant who was once an enthusiastic innovator, which was done, at least in part, by his own colleagues and other doctors involved in management. There are many lessons to be learnt but the crucial one is that this is how not to do it.

People need to be motivated to perform well and to stay in the job; motivation, therefore, is one of the key roles of management. Some of the work on this subject will be considered in the first part of the article as a backdrop to a discussion on a number of practical issues which are directly relevant to doctors in management.

Motivation

After interviews with 200 engineers and accountants in Pittsburgh, United States, in 1966 Herzberg found that five factors were associated with feelings of job satisfaction and that five different factors had the reverse effect[2]:

Motivating and demotivating factors	
Job satisfaction	*Job dissatisfaction*
Achievement	Company policy/administration
Recognition	Supervision
Work itself	Salary
Responsibility	Interpersonal relations
Advancement	Working conditions

Many surveys over the years have supported this work and suggested that people work best if they are given a worthwhile job and are allowed to get on with it. Theories abound, particularly relating to human needs. For instance, Maslow described an ascending hierarchy of needs (modified by Aldefer)—the need for existence, the need to relate to others, and the need for personal growth.[3] The higher order needs are said to be particularly prevalent where people of intelligence and independence are working on challenging problems and they act as strong motivators. McClelland described a different set of need categories which included power, affiliation, and achievement.[4] A large survey he conducted in the United States indicated a particularly strong positive correlation between high need for achievement and high levels of performance.

Handy, however, in describing these theories, questions whether satisfied workers actually work harder, although he believes that they will tend to stay at work and in the same organisation.[5] He argues, on the principle of reinforcement, as many do, that it is incentives which lead individuals to increase their efforts. These are not, of course, related to just money but also include promotion, status, and independence among many others. But Handy points out that incentives are only likely to work if:

• people perceive the increased reward to be worth the extra effort
• the performance can be measured and clearly attributed to the individual
• the individual wants that particular type of reward
• the increased performance will not just become the new minimum standard.

So, getting the best out of people like doctors, must require attention to their individual needs, both for satisfaction and

103

personal growth, and to the sort of rewards that will act as an incentive to them.

Job design

On the basis of his survey work, Herzberg produced a set of principles for job design which included the following:
- remove some controls while retaining accountability
- increase accountability of individuals for their own work
- give the person a complete natural unit of work
- grant additional authority to the employee in his/her own activity
- introduce new and more difficult tasks not previously handled

This type of approach—increasing motivation through increasing individual responsibility—became known as "job enrichment" and has been echoed by several writers. Interestingly, doctors, at least those in the career grades, have had a degree of real professional independence until recent years, their jobs did satisfy most of the above principles, and they were generally well motivated. Unfortunately, the constraints imposed by the NHS changes, the new bureaucracy and, frequently in hospitals, a management style based on control and coercion (McGregor's 'X' Theory) has led to profound demotivation and loss of morale. It is therefore particularly distressing when doctors seek, in addition, to demoralise rather than to motivate their own colleagues.

Well thought out job design is crucial before the advertisement of a post is even considered. Accurate description of jobs, all of which should contribute to an organisation's effectiveness, is fundamental to the development of an efficient staffing system. The job needs to motivate by taking account of the sort of needs described above. Wall confirmed the potential of this type of approach and showed that, when properly implemented, it can benefit both job satisfaction and productivity.[6] However, he also pointed out that to ignore implementation issues, such as organisational structure and practice, is to court disaster.

In the case study there was a clear mismatch between the expectations of the sitting consultants and those of the person appointed. No thought seemed to have been given to how the new role would fit with other activity and the general objectives of the division. Were potential medical colleagues properly consulted about the make up of the job? If not and there was a change that would affect them, it is perhaps not surprising that antagonism developed.

In fact, in this case the job description may have accorded with Herzberg's principles of job design in giving a degree of autonomy to the consultant, but this was then completely undermined in practice, perhaps because the implementation issues were not considered. When expectation is forcibly lowered in this way, demotivation will undoubtedly follow. Full discussion between those involved at an early stage has a better chance of achieving a job description all can agree with and support.

Appointment

To get the best out of a person, the best person for the particular job should be appointed. Some writers, such as Bowen *et al*, suggest that people should be hired to fit the characteristics of the organisation not just the requirements of the job, but an organisational needs analysis to fit every job would make recruitment even more complicated than it is already.[7] Nevertheless, consideration does need to be given to the context of the job as well as the content during the selection process.

As well as a job description it is useful to have a good idea of the sort of person required beforehand. An agreed person specification can help with this, particularly when there are external assessors on the panel. Ideally this should all be agreed before the post is advertised as the advertisement should be founded on a careful analysis of the job itself and aimed at the type of person described in the person specification.

The selection process should aim to:

- attract a sufficiently wide field of suitable candidates
- uphold the organisation's image and reputation
- be fair and be seen to be fair
- observe any constraints imposed by legislation or internal policies

The BMA has produced excellent guidance on good practice in recruitment and selection which, given the increasing scrutiny of appointments procedures, is worth reading.[8] If the wrong person is appointed, as may have happened in the case study, then the consequences can be both serious and long lasting. Medical managers should evaluate appointments for accuracy of job analysis, effectiveness of methods used, and reliability of selectors' judgements but, more particularly, they should ensure that their training policy covers support training for appointment procedures: the investment is well worth it.

Giving feedback

How to encourage improved performance is a much debated subject. The job satisfiers and suggestions for job enrichment above will all help to get the best out of people, but external feedback on performance is also necessary to encourage improvement and, if done properly, can increase motivation. The quasi-disciplinary hearing described in the case study, which was used solely to give destructive feedback, was a complete disaster in relation to motivation and probably did not do a lot for performance either.

Those who oppose formal performance appraisal often cite Deming who stated: "It leaves people bitter, crushed, bruised, battered, desolate, despondent, dejected, feeling inferior, some even depressed, unfit for work for weeks after receipt of rating, unable to comprehend why they are inferior."[9] This can happen particularly when appraisal produces formal performance ratings or is linked to remuneration, but the process need not have these results.

Harper argues for a developmental approach which jointly involves both parties in assessing capabilities and potential, and exploring ways in which performance might be improved.[10] Among other things, this should lead to both becoming aware of requirements for further training and development. A positive and motivating outcome to the exercise can also be encouraged by goal setting, as long as the goals are clear, jointly agreed, and provide a challenge. Locke and Latham have reported that this can lead to improvements in performance ranging from 11% to 27%.[11] But in medicine many seem to find this type of process threatening. There is fierce resistance to appraisal of professional "performance" by lay managers for good reason. But clinical audit is an important type of self appraisal and surely it is time other clinical colleagues—perhaps clinical directors—became involved in giving feedback and agreeing joint goals for the coming year. Peer review is fundamental to medical profession-alism and, with proper training for all parties, annual review and goal setting could lead to increased motivation and to better performance.

Performance appraisal is already a strong feature of general management and if approached correctly medical managers should gain much from it. Apart from the motivational benefits described above, it is a good time to discuss the organisation's overall strategy, identifying how it relates to the manager's area of work and the part to be played in its implementation. It is therefore important for the organisation and the manager in promoting strategic objectives, encouraging involvement, and developing a team approach.

Pay and performance

Herzberg argues that poor pay can lead to job dissatisfaction but does good pay related to "performance" lead to improved satisfaction and better performance? This is a controversial issue and could be the subject of an entire article in itself, but to answer the question, as Kohn argues in an article entitled "Why incentive plans cannot work,"[12] rewards do motivate people, they motivate people to get rewards.

Referring to Handy's four points on making incentives work,[5] the first requires individuals to perceive that the increased reward is worth the effort. Most doctors believe that they are already making a considerable effort across a wide front for the NHS, so performance related pay would probably have to be used to encourage a change in focus or increased effort in specific areas, to the detriment of others. There would have to be very full consultation on this and, even so, it would have to be a high risk management strategy.

This leads on to Handy's second point about the need to be able to measure the performance to be paid extra for and to attribute it fairly. Professional work is notoriously difficult to measure, particularly in relation to effectiveness, and this would be a major stumbling block. It might further discourage the essential "time, touch and compassion" and those crucial activities which are difficult to measure, such as innovation, or leave them dependent on doctors' good will—a fast diminishing commodity. The system would also be seen to be unfair and would lose all credibility if performance was constrained in some way by restriction of the resources required to do the job.

Handy's third point is that the individual has to want the particular reward on offer. When extra pay is the reward there will, of course, be variation from doctor to doctor but certainly, for instance, a substantial number of consultants make a conscious decision not to undertake as much private practice as they could; to them extra pay may not be a great motivator. The final point is that the increased performance should not just become the new minimum standard; this is self evident and would have to be given due weight by managers when change is almost constant in many areas of medicine today.

Bevan and Thompson undertook a wide survey for the Institute of Manpower Studies and found no evidence that improved organisational performance in the private sector is associated with the operation of a formal performance management system.[13] They went on to argue that, using certain approaches, performance management could reinforce a disposition to short termism and set back organisational effectiveness in the long term. They suggest that for performance management to have any success, emphasis is needed on development driven approaches, such as those described in this article, rather than on reward driven models.

Complaints and discipline

This is an area where it is difficult to get the best out of people but where it should be possible to be reasonable and fair to reduce the chance of complete demotivation. Huberman argues that self respect is probably the most potent motivator of satisfactory performance and disciplined behaviour, but also suggests that respect for "management" is an important factor so management must do all it can to gain the respect of those "managed".[14] His article, entitled "Discipline without punishment," describes a 'Y' Theory approach which gives each individual every possible and reasonable chance to play a positive and satisfactory part. The case study gives an example of a different type of approach which, while not common is not unusual and, if there are inadequate safeguards in place, it can happen to anybody if someone in authority develops a personal grudge against them.

A discipline policy should cover two main issues: substandard performance or behaviour and litigation avoidance. There should always be a formal discipline policy and this must be fairly applied; it is particularly important to agree performance standards or determine clearly defined work expectations for each job so that all parties can agree when a variance has occurred.

Gossip and innuendo cannot form the basis of any action and should be stopped, if possible, at source if no formal complaints are to be made. Any person about whom a complaint has been made is entitled to know the nature of the complaint, who has made it, and to be given the opportunity to respond to it. If there is no substance to the complaint the slate should be wiped clean and the doctor informed immediately.

If the doctor needs to be interviewed or counselled then this should either be done one to one, supportively, and in complete confidence, or if a panel of some sort is to be formed the doctor must be given the opportunity of being accompanied by a friend to the hearing; if this is not done it can appear rather like a "kangaroo court." If after this the matter has to be pursued formal procedures should be invoked as these have been designed to ensure fairness to all parties. Again, if there is to be no action then the slate must clearly be wiped clean.

These are sometimes extremely delicate issues and bad handling can lead to long term bitterness and demotivation all round. There are often no easy answers but the general approach should follow the old adage "do as you would be done by."

Training and development

Training and development has to be regarded as central to getting the best out of people. Keep promotes the importance of investment in training and development as a test of whether an organisation is treating its staff as a resource, or as a cost commodity.[15] Organisations that invest in their staff in this way, he argues, will motivate, retain, and develop them to make best use of their skills and maximise the chances of continuous improvement which will lead to continued success.

This is a massive subject which one cannot do justice to here, but, in general, writers in the field would agree that training must not only tie in with the needs of the individual and the needs of the job, but also the needs of the organisation which is providing the investment. In medicine there has always been an emphasis on self development; medical managers or clinical directors should facilitate and encourage this but it should fit with the goals jointly identified in feedback discussion. If it does fit then funding should be almost automatic as it should both motivate and improve performance.

Management training is also essential to enable those doctors involved in management to learn how to get the best out of their colleagues. It should cover all the areas discussed in this article and must include communication, counselling, dealing with complaints and approaches to professional discipline. Unfortunately, in many parts of the NHS there has been an increasing rift between doctors and managers, albeit often promoted by government policies. Both parties need to learn more about each other's philosophies and it may be that more multidisciplinary development work would encourage this. Lack of understanding can lead to antagonism and bitterness which brings out the worst rather than the best in people; more has to be done to change attitudes and encourage cooperation if care of patients is really to be team effort involving and motivating all concerned.

Summary

In summary, to get the best out of people the McGregor Theory 'Y' manager will be supportive and collaborative rather than controlling. The aim will be to appoint staff to properly designed jobs and to motivate them by working with them and agreeing joint goals, by encouraging self development and appropriate training, and by being both firm and fair. In essence this manager will care about colleagues and see them as a resource to be nurtured rather than competitors to be undermined, or as costs to be cut. If the doctor in the case study had been treated in this way perhaps he might still be motivating and treating British patients instead of going to Saudi Arabia where he feels more greatly valued both as an individual and a professional.

Key point summary

- Getting the best from people requires attention to their individual needs

- A well thought out job description and an accurate description of the job are essential

- Feedback can help promote strategic objectives, motivate, and develop team work

- Managers need to encourage self development and to provide appropriate training

- Proper structures for support, complaints, and assessment need to be established

1 McGregor D. *The human side of enterprise.* New York: McGraw-Hill, 1960.
2 Herzberg F. *Work and the nature of man.* Cleveland, Ohio: World Publishing Co, 1966.
3 Maslow A. *Motivation and personality.* New York: Harper and Row, 1954.
4 McClelland DC. *Achievement and entrepreneurship: a longitudinal study.* Cambridge, MA. Harvard University Press, 1963.
5 Handy CB. *Understanding organisations.* London: Penguin Business, 1985.
6 Wall T. 'What's new in job design?' *Personnel Management* 1984; **16**: 27–9.
7 Bowen DE, Ledford GE, Nathan BR. Hiring for the organisation not the job. *Academy of Management Executive* 1991; **5**: 35–51.
8 BMA. Committee on the Career Progress of Doctors. *Guidance for good practice in the recruitment and selection of doctors.* London: BMA, June 1994.
9 Deming WE. *Out of crisis: quality, productivity and competitive position.* Cambridge: Cambridge University Press, 1986.
10 Harper SC. A developmental approach to performance appraisal. *Business Horizons* 1983; **26** (No 5) 68–74.
11 Locke EA, Latham GP. *Goal setting: a motivational technique that works.* London: Prentice Hall, 1984.
12 Kohn A. Why incentive plans cannot work. *Harvard Business Review* 1993; **71** (No 5) 54–63.
13 Bevan S, Thompson M. Performance management at the crossroads. *Personnel Management* 1991; **23**: 37–9.
14 Huberman J. Discipline without punishment. *Harvard Business Review* 1964; **42**: 62–8.
15 Keep E. Corporate training strategies: the vital component. In: Storey J, ed. *New perspectives on human resources management.* London: Routledge, 1989: 109–25.

11 The potential for marketing planning in an NHS trust

MALCOLM McDONALD, CHRISTINE MILES

No planning procedure can predict the future with complete accuracy. None the less those managing NHS trusts, like their counterparts in industry and commerce, must somehow try to anticipate it so as to plan appropriately. This is no easy task at the best of times, but during periods of rapid change and uncertainty, it is even more difficult. Too much is at stake to rely on good fortune or an irreproachable moral stance as being enough to allow an organisation to win through.

Learning theorists claim that we learn through our mistakes. In general the lessons from industry were expensive when it came to planning ahead. Companies have been slow to adopt a marketing approach and those that went under paid the ultimate price. NHS trusts can learn from the collective mistakes which have gone before.

This chapter attempts to remove some of the mystique which surrounds marketing. It will consider some of the marketing tools which are valuable in the preparation of a marketing plan.

What is marketing?

A delegate setting out on one of our courses suggested, to the amusement of his fellow students, that marketing is "...the application of jargon to common sense." He was visibly deflated when we tended to agree with him. As in most professions, practitioners develop a convenient vocabulary which aids communication to insiders, but which is opaque and incomprehensible to everyone else. Marketing, like accounting, and medicine, among others, is equally guilty of this charge. As a result, the "common sense" element has become obscured by a combination of mystery, hyperbole, and banter. Let's put the record straight. Marketing is not about selling, nor is it about parting the gullible and unwary from their hard earned money. It is far more mundane and down to earth. Reduced to basics, marketing is the process of matching the resources of the supplying organisation with identified customers needs, so that both parties achieve their objectives.

Philosophically, this definition does not seem to be very contentious, yet its blandness hides some very important organisational issues. The implications are that: the organisation is clear about its customers and their needs (which is often not the case); it actually wants to satisfy customer needs (as opposed to, say, providing the things it finds easiest to provide, or making profits at all costs, regardless of the consequences); it has the appropriate resources and technology to succeed (which, again, is not always the case).

In an imperfect world it is inevitable that this matching process starts off as something of a compromise. However, by making a decision to base the business on the needs of its users, the organisation can develop the necessary skills, products, and services to ensure that it becomes increasingly attractive to its customers, both actual and potential. This in turn earns it the prospect of justifying further investment. Thus, success feeds on success.

Alternatives to the marketing approach

There are many alternative approaches to marketing. *Technology* is one. The problem is it is often not enough. Indeed, in the United Kingdom few should need reminding of the famous technology breakthroughs that have led to bankruptcy.

Another is *production efficiency*, which focuses on a low cost approach. Alas, this approach eventually fails, because customers become more demanding as choice increases.

Yet another is *financial husbandry*, which in many ways, is similar to production orientation. No one needs reminding of the spectacular failure of once great organisations, deserted by their customers because they failed to pay sufficient attention to their needs.

There seem to be two other alternatives to marketing as a means of moving the organisation forward.

Charismatic leadership

Some organisations can be highly successful with a visionary, entrepreneurial figure at their helm. It is the charismatic drive and leadership which inspires those within the organisation, sometimes against great odds, to follow and succeed. Even so, the "business idea" has to resonate with the times in which it is born.

Such an approach can establish the recurring theme for oganisations to remain successful for years. Witness the great religions of the world, and, more prosaically, many of today's grand companies, which owe their origins to the imagination and single mindedness of their founders. However, charisma, power, and drive are not always enough. Leadership alone cannot carry an idea that is basically flawed, and too often the original concept is overtaken by events. Commercial examples abound.

Incrementalism

As a counterbalance to the "big picture" option provided by charismatic leadership, there is the "one small step at a time" approach, which typifies incrementalism. If growth was experienced in part of the business at, say, 10% for the past two years, the thinking goes, "Let's assume we can do better and aim for 11% this year." In practice this softly softly approach at best only limits damage, because the growth experienced by the organisation might be grossly misrepresenting the real growth potential of the market. Incrementalism, therefore, inhibits the organisation from capitalising on new opportunities and, instead, traps it into reliving its past.

Whereas both of these approaches could be said to appeal to the emotions, the first to "blind faith" and the second to "security," marketing alone brings an analytical and essentially rational dimension to the forward planning conundrum. It is this dimension which sets it apart.

114

Marketing planning

Again, stripped of its obfuscating jargon, marketing planning is a fairly straightforward, four stage process involving the determination of: the strategic context; the situation review; formulation of marketing strategy; and resource allocation and monitoring.

The strategic context:	Specifying what the organisation wants to be and what it wants to be achieving at some time in the future.
The situation review:	Understanding the factors both within and outside the organisation which are going to help or hinder in attaining its ambitions.
Marketing strategy formulation:	Establishing the best mix of products and services to meet the strategic and situational scenario.
Resource allocation and monitoring:	Ensuring that resources are allocated in ways that make the greatest contribution, and checking that this actually happens.

The output of this process, the strategic marketing plan, covering a period of about three years, is a shortish document (probably of no more than 25 pages) that spells out certain criteria:

- the organisation's mission
- a financial summary
- a market summary
- SWOT (strengths, weaknesses, opportunities and threats) analyses on key elements of the market
- a summary of the SWOTs
- overall assumptions
- overall marketing objectives and strategies
- budget details

Establishing the strategic context

The first consideration is to define the organisation so that its sense of purpose and direction is clear to everyone who has a stake in it. For a trust, this means its staff, fundholders, the immediate

115

medical infrastructure and the community it plans to serve. Such a definition is encapsulated in the *mission statement*. Ideally this will not exceed one A4 page and will include the following:

Role There should be a vision of the role towards which the trust is striving—for example, to be a centre of excellence, to be the obvious first choice of anyone in its catchment area, to attract the brightest and best medical staff, etc.

Business definition This should clarify the benefits that the trust provides and the needs it satisfies.

Distinctive competences These are the skills on which any success to date has been founded.

Indications for the future Here the values of the trust are made explicit in terms of what type of work it will, might, and will never undertake.

It is only in the past decade that the value of such a mission statement has become recognised, for, when tackled seriously, it provides a touchstone which can help decision making at all levels. For example, making the choice between two equally valid options can be simplified by considering which is most consistent with the mission statement.

Thus, the mission, business philosophy, statement of intent (call it what you will), should say something unique about the trust which is unlikely to be applicable to any other organisation. Those missions which are mere "window dressing," full of platitudes and pious hopes, serve no real purpose and certainly never engage the hearts and minds of those to whom they are addressed.

Mission statement (Midtown Hospital endocrine and metabolic unit)

To provide treatment of, advice on, and prevention of complications, for a wide range of endocrine and metabolic diseases for the local population. Also to take advantage of the ease of access afforded by the location of the hospital, to attract patient referrals which would otherwise go to hospitals further afield.

To perform relevant clinical research and training for professional staff, in particular to meet the increased training needs of general practitioners as "shared care" for diabetic patients becomes more popular.

To rationalise services that are currently offered so as to provide better value for money.

Having established a sense of personal identity, the next element of the strategic context phase of the marketing plan is to determine what the organisation should actually be achieving some years hence. In industry a three year planning window is widely accepted for quite pragmatic reasons. A longer period is beset with greater uncertainty; a shorter period is not normally adequate to achieve a major strategic shift. In practice the time frame for the strategic marketing plan has to be chosen to be compatible with the nature of the business. For example, three years would be ludicrously short for a company engaged in long term capital projects like the aerospace industry.

For a trust, these corporate objectives will specify the level of funding it will need to be successful. They will also hone the mission statement into clearer business boundaries, covering:

- which services and customer groups (marketing)
- what kind of facilities (logistics)
- the size and character of the workforce (personnel)
- the image the trust wishes to project (to the community, fundholders, its staff, and so on)

Under the new system of purchasers and providers, income flows will tend to be in proportion to the number of procedures carried out over the planning period. Some might regret this change of emphasis by putting money at the heart of what the trust can and cannot do, but realists will recognise that this has always been the case. What is different is that the trust can plan to "earn" its income, rather than relying on receiving an annual injection of government funding, the level of which often bore more relation to the political exigencies of the moment rather than to the needs of the situation. How the Midtown Hospital endocrine and metabolic unit tackled this is shown in fig 11.1.

The marketing plan is concerned with establishing the best mix of health services for the relevant target population served by the trust. In this sense it greatly simplifies the forward planning process by eliminating many complications and distractions which are clearly the remit of other functional areas such as accounts or personnel.

The situation review

The objective of this phase of the marketing planning process is to identify the key factors, both within and outside the trust, which will have a bearing on its fortunes. In an article like this it is

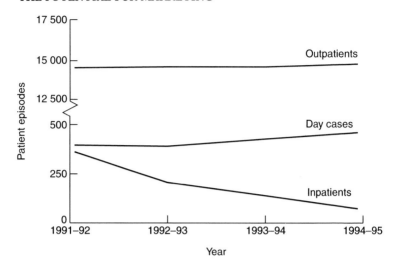

Outpatient attendances	1991–2	1992–3	1993–4	1994–5
Outpatient attendances	14 100	14 250	14 450	14 850
Inpatient episodes	350	220	140	100
Day cases	380	380	420	470

This three year business plan shows a:
5.3% increase in outpatient activity; 26% increase in day cases;
71% decline in inpatient episodes.

Figure 11.1

impossible to go into detail regarding what should be investigated. However, in general terms the trust should be concerned with factors likely to make an impact on it. It is often convenient to group these under four broad headings: the business environment; the market; the competition; the organisation.

The information generated by the situation review does not appear in the marketing plan. Instead it is summarised in the form of a "market" summary, which should be no more than three or four pages long. The purpose is to make it clear to anyone concerned with the plan what the real trends are in the market served by the trust.

The next step is to distil this situation review even more by

118

doing a SWOT analysis (strengths, weaknesses, opportunities and threats) on each of the principal components of the market.

Business environment

- The general economic situation
- Political/legislative changes
- Social/cultural issues
- Technological advances

Market

- Total market and "market share"
- Developments and trends, such as changing demographics
- Market characteristics, such as principal services in the past, volume of demand, patterns of take up, etc.
- Pricing arrangements—normal practice, regulations, etc.
- Channels (how patients are reached, purchasing patterns of fundholders, etc)
- Communications—principal methods of communication, such as direct mail, open days, public relations
- Current best practice, trends, and changes

Competition

- The impact of other trusts which could be construed as being in competition
- Their distinctive competences, business approaches, etc.
- Their pricing policies, efficiency, facilities, etc.
- New entrants, mergers, and acquisitions

Organisation

- Staffing—levels, location, demographic make up, staff turnover, etc.
- Skills and special competences
- Structure or administrative issues
- Bottlenecks and underused facilities
- Patients', staff, and general practitioners' perceptions of the trust

---

Table 11.1 – SWOT on infertility treatment

Critical success factors	Weighting factor	Midtown	Albry	Nearest teaching hospital
Location	10	100	50	50
Ultrasound	10	80	70	70
Facilities (privacy)	20	200	160	120
Success rate (research)	60	480	360	300
Total weighted score	100	860	640	540

An example of one SWOT analysis from Midtown Hospital endocrine and metabolic unit is shown in table 11.1.

The numerical values in the SWOT analysis can be established using independent market research, and techniques are available for establishing what these are. Otherwise, great care is needed to avoid bias. However, it is important to be clear about how "strengths" and "weaknesses" are interpreted, for marketers are more concerned about comparatives rather than absolutes. So a trust is strong if it can outscore a rival on any critical success factor regardless of whether it still has far to go before it could be deemed to be excellent in this area. Its weaknesses must be gauged in a similar way. The completed SWOT analysis provides the input to the next phase of the marketing plan.

Setting marketing objectives and strategies (marketing strategy formulation)

Because the essence of marketing is getting products and services to customers, it follows that marketing objectives can only fall into the categories illustrated in fig 11.2.

A Providing existing services to existing customers;
B providing new services to existing customers;
C providing existing services to new customers;
D providing new services to new customers.

It is box A which provides the basis for the marketing planner; all others introduce an element of the unknown—that is to say, risk. Box D is clearly the most risky option of all.

A technique known as gap analysis can be used to determine the nature of the chosen marketing objectives. Gap analysis allows the

C U S T O M E R S			
	Existing	A	B
	New	C	D
		Existing	New
		Products and Services	

Figure 11.2 Marketing objectives

user to set the required objective, for a future time period, project the likely outcome (given current policies), and then attempt to fill the gap by means of one or more of the following: productivity improvements; better results from current activities; or new activities (either from new services provided, from new users, or from a combination of these). Figure 11.3 illustrates this theory. Figure 11.4 illustrates how this operated in an example from Midtown hospital.

There was a 17.7% increase in productivity over one year

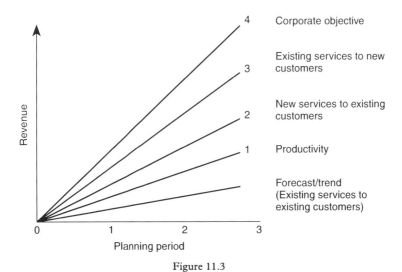

Figure 11.3

(1990–91) due to more efficient management of the clinics. With this efficiency drive expected to continue and a reduction in the number of non-attenders (currently 21% of clinic appointments), it was anticipated that a further 10% increase in productivity could be achieved over the next three years.

By 1994–95 the outpatient workload for osteoporosis treatment will be 915 attendances a year. These patients will be largely from the Midtown market (fig 11.4).

In the context of the situation review it is possible to calculate the revenue to be derived from providing the current range of services to existing customers. In fig 11.4 this reaches level 1, which falls short of the corporate objective. By tightening up in various ways, the initial prediction could be revised to point 2, thus closing the original gap through productivity. Even so, the predicted results still fall short of their target and more must be done to close this strategic gap.

Often, the next best choice is to provide new services for existing customers, because it is often quicker and easier to introduce new procedures than to find new customers (but this will not always be the case for trusts).

Another implication of introducing this strategy is that the trust

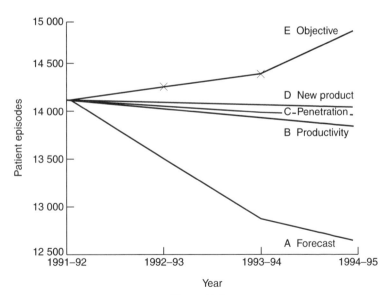

Figure 11.4

has the appropriate skills and resources to provide new services which are required. If not it must pursue the next strategy option of finding new customers for its existing range of services. Finally, a combination of both new services and new customers may be required.

By focusing on opportunities from the SWOT analysis and playing to its strengths, the trust can follow the best options that present themselves, while at the same time achieving its coporate objectives.

Gap analysis is a comparatively simple, yet essential, technique for deciding on a range of marketing objectives (fig 11.4).

The 80/20 rule

As with other types of business, there will always be some minority products or services which in themselves are not profitable, yet, which, for various reasons, must still be provided. Is there still room for these in a marketing plan? The short answer is yes, as long as the rest of the business is managed efficiently. The justification for this is: empirically, 20% of services generate 80% of costs; if management attention focuses on these 20%, costs can be contained and revenues maximised, thereby enabling other minority activities to be undertaken; investment in such minority products or services should be kept to a minimum.

Ideally, it should be known how each product or service contributes to the whole output of the trust. In this way it becomes possible to manage the range of activities as a complete portfolio, rather than as a set of unconnected services.

Portfolio management

Every service or product can be plotted on a "map" and a sense of their direction can be established. The "map", or "directional policy matrix" as it is often referred to is constructed as shown in fig 11.5.

It assumes that any organisation, regardless of its sphere of activity, will not be equally proficient at providing every service it offers, nor will its customer groups all be equally attractive. How the organisation chooses to define these two parameters is a matter

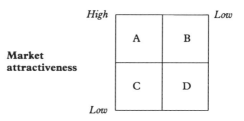

Figure 11.5 Directional policy matrix

of personal choice, For a trust, the following factors could be pertinent (box).

Attractiveness

Little competition
Not price sensitive
High procedure success rates
Few complications

Minimal inpatient content
Growth area (to justify investment)

Strengths

Highly competent at procedures
Compatible with resources
Reputation
Good relationship with main fundholders
Quality standards
Calibre of staff, etc, etc.

By weighing the relative importance of these factors, a procedure can be devised whereby each service or procedure can be "scored" in terms of market attractiveness and its "fit" with organisational strengths.

Each service the trust provides can be plotted on this map by drawing a circle at the intersection of the scores on the vertical and horizontal axes. The circle size should be proportional to the level of funding which that particular service generates. Thus at a glance the relative value and positioning of all services can be accommodated. The reason for doing this will become clear in a moment, when the meaning of each "box" on the matrix is explained.

Box A represents the key services and procedures for which the trust is likely to develop a widespread reputation. Not only is the market attractive in the trust's eyes, but the trust is also well matched to provide whatever is required.

124

Box B represents newer services or procedures which have been introduced because of the higher market attractiveness score, but for which the organisation has yet to develop sufficient strengths.

Box C also reflects a high compatibility with the trust's strengths, but here the attractiveness score is much lower. This means that some of the resources expended on these services might be used more productively on those which feature in box A. Items in this box might represent yesterday's "stars" which have become less attractive.

Box D is clearly a dubious area for any services or procedures, because not only is the market unattractive, but also the trust is using few of its strengths. Ideally items which are located in the box might be better provided by another trust for whom these could be Box A items—that is, another trust could view the market differently and would certainly have different strengths.

In simple terms a general strategy is identified by each box on the directional policy matrix as follows:

Box A Promote expertise (invest in resources and communications).

Box B Develop strengths (therefore invest selectively in personnel and the organisation.

Box C Do not actively seek new customers or use up too many vital resources (monitor costs).

Box D Seek to withdraw or subcontract the work elsewhere, or, at least, minimise costs if these are services you must provide.

Figure 11.6 shows not only how the portfolio of services is perceived today, but also how it is planned to be developed at Midtown Hospital. (The new circles indicate future positioning.) This example shows that the diabetes market will become more attractive because of increased screening for diabetes. The strengths will be increased with the implementation of the "shared care" model and the diabetes centre. There will be a greater demand for infertility services and the endocrine and metabolic unit will gain market share from its competitors.

Resource allocation, budgeting, and monitoring

In many ways the most difficult part of the marketing planning process is stage 3, where high quality conceptual thinking is required to set objectives and formulate strategies. However, this will all be to no avail unless resources are allocated sensibly to allow

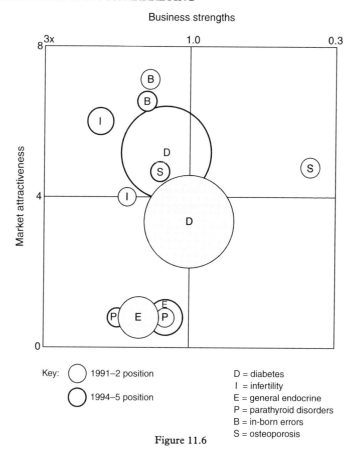

Figure 11.6

the organisational thinking to be converted into reality (figs 11.7 and 11.8).

There will be penetration of the Midtown market for the treatment of diabetes, general endocrine and metabolic, infertility and calcium disorders. For diabetes, this will be achieved through the establishment of a diabetic centre and a "shared care" model, which will be promoted through educational programmes to general practitioners. For calcium disorders, this market penetration will be achieved by repositioning the existing service to include the treatment of osteoporosis. All the services will be promoted to general practitioners in the homemarket and priced, if allowed, at a discount.

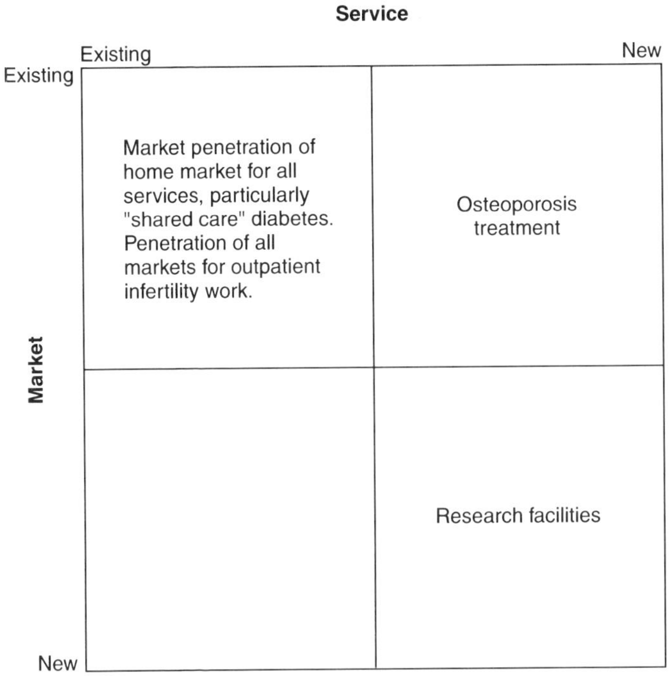

Service

Existing   New

Figure 11.7

For infertility services, market penetration across all the markets will be achieved by increasing the number of referrals from existing customers and expanding the hospital's customer base in obstetrics and gynaecology hospital departments. Results of the market research work will be distributed to these departments.

There will be a transfer of inpatient treatment to day case treatment. This will follow on from careful analysis of clinical practice.

The spare capacity on the endocrine and metabolic unit will be used for medical research performed by other clinical teams and the bays in ward will be sponsored by pharmaceutical companies.

Financial projections

The major changes in costs are presented below:

1992-3: £5000 for the upgrade of outpatient facilities to

127

Outpatient attendances

Market	1991–92	1992–93	1993–94	1994–95
Diabetes	5046	5046	5046	5046
Infertility	1221	1290	1410	1471
Paediatrics	3261	3265	3265	3265
General endocrine	2998	2932	2866	2800
Parathyroid/ calcium	1233	1159	1085	1011
Inborn errors	341	341	341	341
Subtotal	14 100	14 033	14 013	13 934
Osteoporosis		217	937	916
Total	14 100	14 250	14 450	14 850

Inpatient episodes

Thompson	685	38	25	20
Carroll	545	37	25	17
Creaser	31	21	14	10
O'Neill	42	19	18	15
Scott	155	105	58	38
Total	350	220	140	100

Day cases

Thompson	39	43	47	60
Carroll	274	210	180	160
Creaser	21	27	27	35
O'Neill	22	23	28	30
Scott	24	52	78	100
Subtotal	380	355	360	385
Osteoporosis*	0	25	60	85
Total	380	380	420	470

*New work carried out by a clinical assistant appointed in 1992–93

Figure 11.8

produce a diabetic centre. A reduction in medical staff by one senior house officer (£24 780).

1993-4: A reduction in medical staff by one registrar (£27 200) but an increase by one clinical assistant (£25 000).

1994-5: An appointment of one clinical assistant (£25 000).

Sponsorship for the operating costs of the endocrine and metabolic unit could be obtained from the pharmaceutical industry. This will be about £82 000 a year plus any chemical pathology variable costs.

External communications

We do not intend to elaborate on the details of strategy here, because we believe that readers will be familiar with what is involved. Having said this, there will be one area for consideration that would be unlikely to feature in other planning approaches. This is the area of external communications. In order to influence markets, it is important to communicate with them (fig 11.9). Normally this is achieved in two ways: (a) through personal transactions—face to face; by telephone; or by letter, or (b) by impersonal methods—advertising; and public relations.

The objective of any communications programme is to influence members of a target market

It cannot necessarily be assumed that everyone automatically

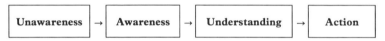

Figure 11.9 The communication chain

knows what the trust is capable of providing most effectively. Therefore, they must be encouraged to approach the trust for help. Thus an integrated communication "plan" must be devised (with budgets) directed essentially at fundholding general practitioners, purchasing consortia, consultants and the relevant areas of the local community. Such is the power and potential of communications, it cannot be left to chance, nor starved of resources.

Conclusions

Regardless of the political dimension of the recent changes in the NHS and the speed of their introduction, health provision has always been subject to the laws of supply and demand. In the past it was the former which dominated, but now the new approach purports to put demand in the forefront. Just how far the NHS becomes customer driven remains to be seen. However, it is clear that those in management positions in self determining trusts must learn more about marketing planning if their organisations are to succeed.

If our experience in industry is anything to go by it is not easy for an organisation to switch suddenly to a marketing oriented culture, especially when marketing itself is viewed as the equivalent of the golden horde of Gengis Khan battering at the frontiers of Christendom. We have found that it can take up to three years before a strategic marketing system can be fully implemented, because what might seem glaringly obvious is fraught with practical problems.

First, as we have indicated, it is a matter of engendering the right attitudes throughout the trust. Then, information systems need to be devised to provide the right inputs. Then a suitable plan for introducing the planning has to be developed. Who does what has to be established, and so on, and all this has to be done against a background of the normal and busy work routine.

Not least of the problems is that top management often pay lip service to marketing planning without ever being fully committed. Their "semidetached" stance inevitably causes a cynical antimarketing undercurrent in the organisation, which is ultimately the death knell to any meaningful initiative. Thus marketing planning is more than a cognitive process, for it profoundly and irreversibly affects the organisational infrastructure. To become customer focused or driven is not a new piece of management jargon, but a statement of intent. It is a declaration that the organisation will stop contemplating its own navel and, instead, learn how to enter into a mutually beneficial relationship with the community it chooses to serve.

Key point summary

- If a business is based on the needs of its customers it can develop the necessary skills, products, and services, justifying further investment during the process

- Marketing planning is a four stage process involving the determination of strategic context, situation review, formulation of marketing strategy, and resource allocation

- An integrated communication plan (with budgets) will effectively "market" services to general practitioners, purchasing consortia, and the local community

- It can take up to three years before a strategic marketing system is fully implemented

12 Decision analysis for medical managers

JG THORNTON, RJ LILFORD

Case study

The obstetricians at "Enterprise Hospital Trust" in the northern city of Yeeds are trying to persuade the health authority to buy serum screening for Down's syndrome for all pregnant women in the district.[1] The director of purchasing was about to approve this when she received a letter from Lady Pressure, chair of the community health council. Lady Pressure's grandchild had just died of congenital toxoplasmosis, and she wondered why this screening was not offered in Yeeds. She enclosed literature from the Toxoplasmosis Trust calling for a screening programme, and reminded the manager that screening had been offered in France for years. Why was Yeeds so backward? Finally, the manager herself was aware that the recent identification of the cystic fibrosis gene made screening for that disease technically simple.

The right decision in this case is not obvious. It is tempting to choose the cheapest programme, but perhaps a slightly more expensive one will produce greater health gain. This itself is difficult to measure, and different programmes do not simply save different numbers of lives. How can we compare prevention of the birth of a baby with Down's syndrome with the birth of a baby with cystic fibrosis? Each programme will also have other "costs": they will cause some miscarriages and make quite a lot of parents anxious.

Typically, managers resolve such conflicts by reference to previous practice, to what others do and by subjectively evaluating the claims of the various pressure groups. The problem with such political methods is that "he who shouts loudest" is likely to win, without necessarily being the most deserving. Sometimes decision makers will want to stand back and attempt a more thoughtful analyis.

Decision analysis

Decision analysis is a way of doing this by analysing the benefits and harms systematically, so that the trade offs are explicit.[2] Business people often use it[3] and much of the literature refers to their problems.[4] An increasing amount of published data concerns health management problems such as neonatal intensive care of very low birthweight infants[5] or colposcopy.[6] The conclusions are often surprising. The marginal cost of preventing one death from bowel cancer using the recommended policy of measuring a sixth faecal occult blood sample was estimated at US 47 million dollars in 1975.[7] Screening for ovarian cancer increases women's life expectancy by an average of one day.[8]

We live in a political world and wise managers will rarely decide solely on the basis of decision analysis. Nevertheless, it will inform their final decision and provide a powerful means to defend it. Those who dislike formal methods must recognise that there is little rational alternative within a planned health care system. Individual planners may wish to follow their own intuitions when they make decisions, but they can hardly expect others to accept that method. A market, with many consumers deciding how to spend their health care money, would be sensitive to more factors than those which comprise decision analysis,[9] but it may not provide the equity which current health care systems seek.

Decision analysis is the application to decision making of the

> *The spirit of decision analyis is divide and conquer. Decompose a complex problem into simpler problems, get your thinking clear on these simpler problems, paste these analyses together with logical glue, and come out with a program for action for the complex problem. Experts are not asked complicated fuzzy questions, but crystal clear, unambiguous, elemental, hypothetical questions.*
>
> Raiffa 1968[10]

reductionist approach that has been so successful elsewhere in science.

Clinical decisions

Clinical decision analysis usually guides treatment for an individual. Consider a woman wondering whether to undergo amniocentesis for the prenatal diagnosis of spina bifida. After measurement of serum α fetoprotein and an ultrasound scan her residual risk has been estimated to be 1 in 200.[11] However, amniocentesis carries a small risk of miscarriage (fig 12.1) and the correct course also depends on the *disutility* to her of having an affected child or losing a normal pregnancy. We measure these by a series of lotteries (fig 12.2). For the individual to whom a 25% chance of spina bifida and pregnancy termination is equal, we say that the disutility of termination is 0.25 on a scale where a normal baby is 0 and spina bifida 1. The course of minimum expected disutility is calculated by multiplying probabilities and disutilities.

In our examples we measure *dis*utility rather than utility as most people find this easier when the bad outcomes of miscarriage

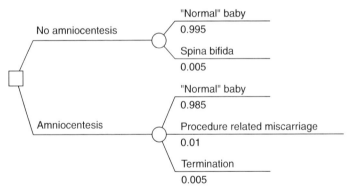

Figure 12.1 Decision tree for amniocentesis for spina bifida. The term "normal" baby is used to indicate an unaffected child. Although many other abnormalities may occur, these will be equally distributed between the two arms of the decision tree. The expected disutility of no amnioscentesis is disutility of spina bifida × probability of spina bifida—$0.005 \times 1 = 0.005$. The expected disutility of amniocentesis is (disutility of procedure related miscarriage × probability of miscarriage) plus (disutility of termination × probability of termination)—$(0.25 \times 0.01) + (0.25 \times 0.005) = 0.00375$. The expected disutility of undergoing amniocentesis is thus less than that of not doing so, and the patient should choose amniocentesis.

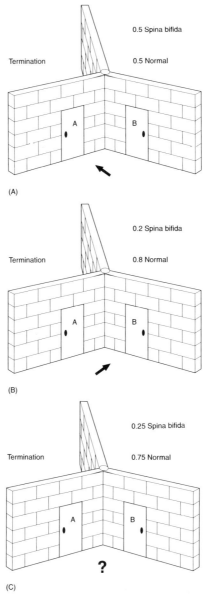

Figure 12.2 A–C The lotteries for the spina bifida decision. For simplicity we assume that the disutility of procedure related miscarriage is equal to that of termination. A second lottery could be performed if these were significantly different.

or handicap are less frequent than the good ones. We use disutility rather than the more euphonious term cost to avoid confusion with monetary costs.

Analysis of management decisions

The above example is concerned with helping an individual, but managers can use the same techniques to decide for groups. It is easy enough to calculate the relevant probabilities, but difficult to include utilities because there is no generally accepted way of measuring these for groups, and few empiric data. Nevertheless, managers have to make decisions, and in doing so an assessment of population utilities is implied—whether or not it is made explicit.

Let us perform population decision analyses for screening for Down's syndrome, congenital toxoplasmosis, and cystic fibrosis. To keep things simple, we focus on the outcomes affected by screening, and ignore background rates of disability and miscarriage. In all three examples we refer to a hypothetical population of 100 000 pregnancies. We consider first the probabilities of each outcome. Next we compare the disutilities of these outcomes and combine these with the probabilities. Lastly, we discuss monetary costs.

The probabilities of the various outcomes

Screening for Down's syndrome

Without screening 100 babies with Down's syndrome would be born.[12] Assuming an 80% uptake for the screening test and a 75% uptake of amniocentesis with risks of over 1 in 250, 80 000 women would undergo screening and 4000 would screen positive; 3000 would under amniocentesis of whom 30 would miscarry a normal baby. In the process 40 Down's syndrome babies would be detected and the pregnancies aborted (fig 12.3).

Congenital toxoplasmosis screening

A screening programme would involve serial maternal blood tests in pregnancy to identify women who seroconvert, fetal blood sampling to confirm fetal infection, and either antibiotic treatment or abortion of infected fetuses. At best, screening would prevent the birth of 10 disabled babies, for the disutility of 10 terminations and five miscarriages.[13] At worst, the birth of only one disabled baby would be prevented for the disutility of 40

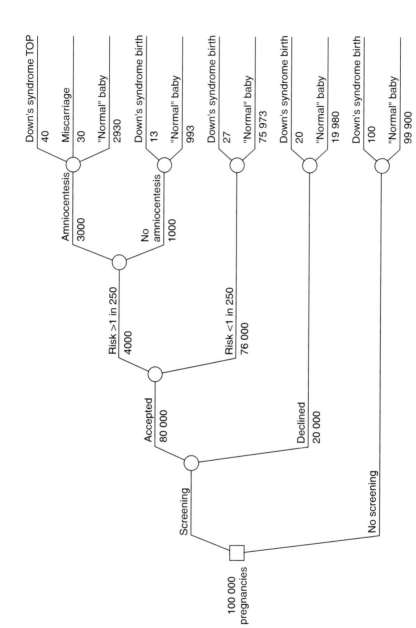

Figure 12.3 The decision tree for Down's syndrome screening for a population of 100 000 pregnancies.

terminations and 12 miscarriages.[14] This uncertainty is one reason why toxoplasmosis screening is not generally offered in the United Kingdom. For the present we will make a "best guess" and assume that five miscarriages related to the procedure and 20 terminations would be caused, to prevent the birth of five babies with congenital toxoplasmosis (decision tree not shown).

Cystic fibrosis screening

Without screening some 40 babies would be born with cystic fibrosis. In a typical programme women would be offered carrier testing first, and their partners would be tested to see if they were positive. Carrier couples would have a one in four risk of having an affected child and would be offered invasive testing. Typically 80 women would undergo amniocentesis or chorionic villus sampling, one would miscarry, and 20 babies with cystic fibrosis would be identified (decision tree not shown).[15]

To decide whether such screening programmes give a net health gain we need to know not only the risks but also the relative disutilities to typical women of the loss of a normal baby, and the birth of a child with Down's syndrome, congenital toxoplasmosis, or cystic fibrosis. We also need to measure the anxiety caused by the programme.

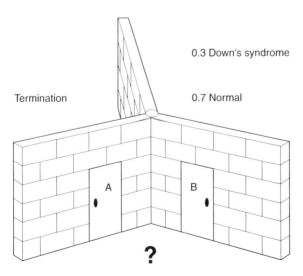

Figure 12.4 Lottery for measuring the relative disutilities of termination or miscarriage and Down's syndrome.

137

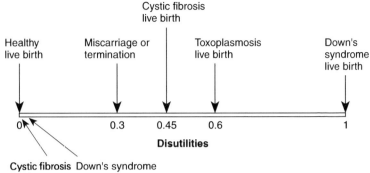

Figure 12.5 Diagram of the disutilities used in the present analyses. Only the disutility of miscarriage or termination and Down's syndrome are based on empiric data. The disutilities of toxoplasmosis and cystic fibrosis and the anxiety of being screen positive seem plausible but have not been formally measured.

Down's syndrome disutilities

Samples of women have performed the relevant lotteries[16] [17] and miscarriage or termination typically has a disutility of about 0.3 on a scale where full health is 0 and Down's syndrome is 1 (figs 12.4 and 12.5). The expected disutility of a screening programme is thus:

70 miscarriages or terminations × 0.3 = 23;

that of not screening is:

40 Down's × 1 (disutility of Down's) = 40.

Screening provides a net gain of 17 "utility units."

One source of error in this calculation is the accuracy of the population utilities used. We have used the medians of possibly unrepresentative samples because these are all that are available. As population health utility surveys, such as the Oregon experiment,[18] become more widespread, representative mean utilities may become available and would be preferable.

Decision analysis is unashamedly utalitarian. It cannot select the correct course of action for people who wish to follow other ethical principles. Those who follow the rule that all human life is sacred from conception onwards will not agree with us, and our analysis ignores their views except in so far as the socially derived utilities take them into account.

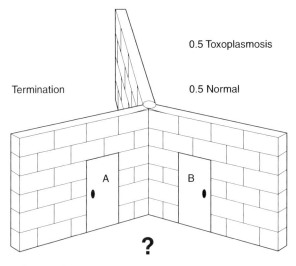

Figure 12.6 Lottery for measuring the relative disutility of termination or miscarriage and toxoplasmosis.

Toxoplasmosis utility

Like the risks, the disutility of having a child with congenital toxoplasmosis is less well defined than that of Down's syndrome.

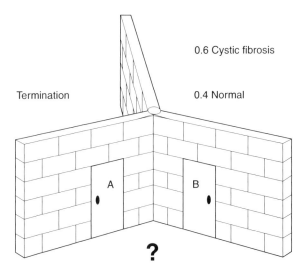

Figure 12.7 Lottery for measuring the relative disutility of termination or miscarriage and cystic fibrosis.

The disease varies in severity, from mild to severe developmental delay, and the more severely affected cases may not survive long. Toxoplasmosis may therefore be of less disutility than Down's syndrome, with a typical life expectancy of 55 years. For our illustration we will assume that toxoplasmosis has only twice the disutility of miscarriage or termination—that is, that people would be indifferent between abortion and a 50% risk of congenital toxoplasmosis (fig 12.6). This corresponds to a disutility of 0.6 (fig 12.7). The "best guess" toxoplasmosis screening programme thus has an expected disutility of:

25 miscarriages or termination $\times$ 0.3;

not screening a disutility of:

five affected babies $\times$ 0.6 (disutility of toxoplasmosis) = 3.

Screening, far from increasing utility, decreases it by 5.3 units.

If the figures on which an analysis is based are uncertain it may be wise to repeat the analysis with different but still plausible risks to see if the best decision changes on sensitivity analysis. A toxoplasmosis screening programme might only cause 15 miscarriages or terminations for every 10 affected births prevented. In that case screening would have a disutility of $15 \times 0.3 = 5$ units, while not screening would have a disutility of $10 \times 0.6 = 6$ units. It seems that even under the most favourable assumptions toxoplasmosis screening adds only marginal value to the community.

Cystic fibrosis utility

There are few data on the disutility of cystic fibrosis, although it is probably perceived as less severe than Down's syndrome and perhaps, because the brain is not affected, as less severe than toxoplasmosis. Let us assume that women on average would be indifferent between a 60% risk of cystic fibrosis and abortion or miscarriage (fig 12.7), corresponding to a cystic fibrosis disutility of 0.45 (fig 12.5). The expected disutility of not screening is thus:

20 cystic fibrosis $\times$ 0.45 = 9;

that of screening is:

21 miscarriages or terminations $\times$ 0.3 = 7.

The screening programme increases utility by 2 units.

The analysis so far suggests that both screening for Down's syndrome and cystic fibrosis increase expected utility, the former more so, while toxoplasmosis screening decreases utility.

The anxiety caused by screening

Much public concern about screening is based on the anxiety it causes to many compared with the good it might do for a few. Even a verbal offer to screen will induce some anxiety, and being screened positive, even if ultimately diagnosed as negative, will cause still more.[19] This anxiety should be debited to the screening programme. The first step is to measure the extent and duration of anxiety, and the second task is to put it onto our utility scale. In the absence of empiric data let us assume that the anxiety caused by being positive for Down's syndrome by screening is such that 1000 women made anxious may be traded off against the prevention of one child with Down's syndrome being born (fig 12.8), and that the anxiety of being a cystic fibrosis carrier is half this because of the lesser severity of the disease. The analysis would go as follows.

In 100 000 pregnancies 4000 women would be rendered anxious because of a "screen positive" test result for Down's syndrome. This is equivalent to $4000 \times 0.001 = 4$ Down's syndrome units. This is added to the other disutilities of screening, 23 units, to make a total disutility of 27 units. This is still outweighed by the prevention of 40 units by screening.

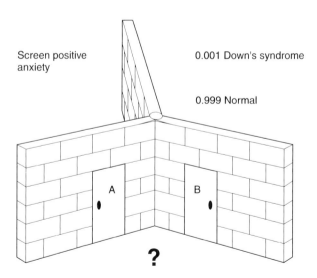

Figure 12.8 Lottery for measuring the disutility of "screen positive" anxiety in terms of a Down's syndrome birth.

Screening for cystic fibrosis would render 5000 women anxious (5000 × 0.0005 = 2.5 units) to be added to the 7 units from miscarriage or termination, making a total disutility of 9.5 units from screening to prevent 9 units from disability. The decision is finely balanced for cystic fibrosis screening, with the conclusion being sensitive to the anxiety of being a carrier, something we do not pretend to know. However, as more managers use decision analysis, these issues will be thrown into sharper focus, and we anticipate that instead of just measuring anxiety, psychologists will in future ask what it means in benefits that should be forgone.

Financial costs

Finally, managers will want a successful screening programme to produce more health gain than the other possible uses for available resources. Toxoplasmosis screening definitely fails on this count. It must cost some money, and as it reduces expected utility, should not be performed. Screening for Down's syndrome and cystic fibrosis add value but do not necessarily add as much as other activities. Screening for Down's syndrome probably provides more utility per pound than most other health interventions because, if we take into account the cost of caring for the Down's syndrome babies whose birth is prevented, it may even save money.[12] If not, we could cost the programmes and turn the decision analysis into a cost–utility analysis. This places all health gains or losses on a universal scale so that the programme under investigation can be compared with any other. In our examples we used "disutility of Down's syndrome" scale and

---

Key point summary

- When doctors treat patients good outcomes must be traded off against bad, taking into account the values of the individuals involved; in management the perceptions of the community as a whole determine the values

- Decision analysis is a way to separate the treatments which add net value from those that do not, and to compare the relative value of beneficial treatments, on the assumption that it might not be possible to implement them all

- It is a powerful means of defending decisions taken, and can be applied to individuals and groups

placed all other disutilities on this. The most popular universal utility scale is the quality adjusted life year (QALY). In principle the prevention of a Down's syndrome birth could be expressed in QALYs and then the utility of screening could be compared pound for pound with any other activity.

1 Wald NJ, Cuckle HS, Densem JW, Nanchahal K, Royston P, Chard T, *et al*. Maternal serum screening for Down's syndrome in early pregnanyc. *BMJ* 1988; **297**: 883-7.
2 Thornton JG, Lilford RJ, Johnson N. Decision analysis in medicine. *BMJ* 1992; **304**: 1099-103.
3 Anonymous. Management brief; risk and reward. *The Economist* 1989; 119-20.
4 French S. *Decision theory. An introduction to the mathematics of rationality*. Chichester: Ellis Horwood, 1988.
5 Boyle MH, Torrance GW, Sinclair JC, Horwood SP. Economic evaluation of neonatal intensive care of very-low-birth-weight infants. *N Engl J Med* 1983; **308**: 1330-7.
6 Johnson N, Sutton J, Thornton JG, Lilford RJ, Johnson VA, Peel KR. Decision analysis for best management of mildly dyskaryotic smear. *Lancet* 1993; **342**: 91-6.
7 Neuhauser D, Lewicki AM. What do we gain from the sixth stool guiac? *N Engl J Med* 1975; **293**: 226-8.
8 Shapira MM, Matchar DB, Young MJ, The effectiveness of ovarian cancer screening. A decision analysis model. *Ann Int Med* 1993; **118**: 838-43.
9 Hayek FA. *The constitution of liberty*. Chicago: University of Chicago Press, 1960.
10 Raiffa H. Decision analysis: introductory lectures on choices under uncertainty. Reading, Massachusetts: Addison-Wesley, 1968: 271.
11 Thornton JG, Lilford RJ, Newcombe RG. Tables for estimation of individual risks of fetal neural tube and ventral wall defects, incorporating prior probability, maternal serum alhafetoprotein and ultrasound examination results. *Am J Obstet Gynecol* 1991; **164**: 154-60.
12 Sheldon TA, Simpson J. Appraisal of a new scheme for prenatal screening for Down's syndrome. *BMJ* 1991; **302**: 1133-6.
13 Stray-Pedersen B. Toxoplasmosis in pregnancy. *Baillière's Clin Obstet Gynaecol* 1993; 7: 107-37.
14 Peckham C, Hall S, Patel N, Hudson C, Rudd P, Joynson D, *et al*. *Prenatal screening for toxoplasmosis in the UK*. Report of a working group. London: Royal College of Obstetricians and Gynaecologists, 1992.
15 Mennie ME, Gilfillan A, Compton M, Curtis L, Liston WA, Pullen I, *et al*. Prenatal screening for cystic fibrosis. *Lancet* 1992; **304**: 214-6.
16 Pauker SP, Pauker SG. The amniocentesis decision: ten years of decision analytic experience. Birth defects; original article series. *March of Dimes Birth Defects Foundation* 1987; **23**: 151-69.
17 Thornton JG, Lilford RJ. Prenatal diagnosis of Down's syndrome; a method for measuring the consistency of women's decisions. *Med Decis Making* 1990; **10**: 288-93.
18 Eddy DM. What's going on in Oregon? *JAMA* 1991; **266**: 417-20.
19 Marteau TM. Psychological costs of screening. *BMJ* 1989; **300**: 1527.

13 Using information for managing clinical services effectively

TIM SCOTT, P JACKSON

Case study

The first report of the Audit Commission suggested that cases suitable for day surgery were being treated inefficiently.[1] Huddersfield featured well below the median for the percentage of those procedures that were performed as day cases. This prompted a local review.

One of the procedures was dilatation and curetterage (D and C). The Audit Commission suggested that 86% of these should be performed as day cases despite the fact that fewer than 50% of these were being performed as day cases in half the districts surveyed. Huddersfield was stated to have a rate of 32%. The gynaecological clinical audit group carried out an initial review using information from the computerised clinial information systm of all D and C procedures performed during the previous two years. The audit meetings are attended by all medical staff working in the department and are open to nurses, nurse managers, and medical students. They are chaired by a consultant who is also the gynaecological representative on the clinical directorate.

A total of 966 cases of D and C had been carried out in the two years. The survey revealed that 23.5% of the patients were under the age of 35 years (fig 13.1). The most common presenting symptom was excessive or frequent menstrual losses (38% of all cases), with irregular bleeding, intermenstrual bleeding, and infertility being other less common symptoms. None of the patients under the age of 50 had malignant disease. Even in patients presenting with postmenopausal bleeding only 12.1% had either malignant disease (adenomatous or squamous carcinoma) or potentially premalignant changes (atypical endometrial hyperplasia) (fig 13.2).

The clinicians agreed that a D and C was essentially a diagnostic test and that its most vital role was in the detection of malignant or premalignant disease. For many of the patients, therefore, it was an unnecessary procedure. There were two alternatives:

(i) patients did not need the test and could begin appropriate treatment for their symptoms; (ii) the histological information could be obtained more simply from a Vabra endometrial biopsy specimen (an outpatient procedure).

Both of the alternatives would improve the quality of care by preventing patients from having to have a general anaesthetic and be admitted to hospital. Treatments of the presenting symptoms could also be started much earlier by eliminating the wait for the D and C to be performed. The numbers of patients placed on the waiting lists would be decreased, thus improving the efficiency of the department. It was agreed that greater selectivity of cases was required. Criteria were then established which the clinicians felt were safe and represented good practice. (The need for such a review has recently been suggested).[2]

The following standards were set:

(i) with rare exceptions D and C is not justified in patients under 35; (ii) D and C should not be performed in patients under 45 unless for irregular bleeding.

These were incorporated in the department handbook of guidelines given to all members of the medical staff. An additional comment advised: "Always consider the possibility of a Vabra as an outpatient procedure." It was also agreed that when a D and C was required, the aim should be to do it as a day case.

Twelve months of data were collected and the situation then reviewed by the gynaecological clinical audit group to see whether the standards had been met. During the year there had been 344 cases in which a D and C was the main procedure, and all but one had been performed as day cases. The patients ($n = 18$) under the age of 35 were now largely limited to those treated by one consultant (fig 13.3). and represented a considerable reduction in numbers from previous years.

Of the patients under 45 years of age who had undergone a D and C, there were 65.4% with excessive or frequent periods, a category felt not to warrant a D and C. One patient with irregular bleeding had atypical endometrial hyperplasia but there were no other sinister histology reports.

The results confirmed the validity of the standards. However, they were not being universally applied. To encourage greater compliance another review was planned after a further 12 months. On that occasion there would be an individual case review with the responsible consultant having to justify the management of each patient that failed to conform to the standards.

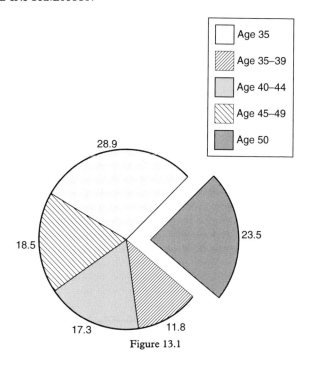

Figure 13.1

Learning points from the case study

Quality of care

Motivation to change clinical services should be driven primarily by a desire to improve the quality of service and not merely to make financial savings. One of the main objectives in managing a clinical service effectively is to strive continually to improve the quality of care. Quality and efficiency are closely linked in that good quality care is both effective and cost efficient medicine. Getting it right first time saves the costs involved in the management of complications—extra drugs, extra investigations, extra theatre visits, re–admissions, and so on. It also prevents additional suffering and prolonged incapacity in the patient.

Information exchange

Information represents a key resource to those managers or clinicians who feel that change is needed to improve the service. Establishing a rational framework for discussion of personal issues

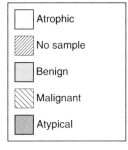

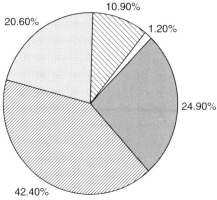

Figure 13.2

of clinical practice helps to defuse some of the natural defensiveness. An environment in which information is shared is a prerequisite for tackling issues of effective clinical practice in an atmosphere of positive cooperation.

The stimulus for change will come from many sources and often, as in the case study, from outside the unit. In this example the response was, perhaps, not what might have been expected. However, the results achieved a substantial improvement in the service provided and in efficiency, because the clinicians had sound information on which to base their managerial actions. The management structure gave the clinicians both the responsibility for ensuring a quality service and also the authority to implement changes. Once these were agreed, the clinicians could then monitor their effects. One of the major benefits of giving doctors the authority to manage is that they are in a unique position to bridge the gap between medical audit and resource management. Close integration of these two processes is imperative for the delivery of a high quality clinical service.

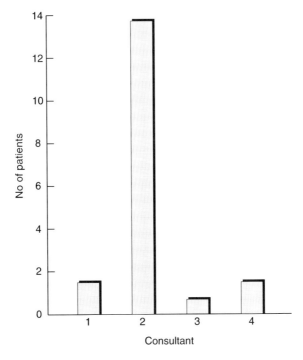

Figure 13.3

The case study clearly shows both how local ownership of data and data retrieval with analysis facilities helped clinical staff to improve the quality of their service. The information systems are relatively simple, but the ability to search the patient database and create a listing of all the patients who had had a D and C was a vital data retrieval step. A specific study could then be conducted on those case notes, using information chosen for the hypothesis under consideration.

In many hospitals the reaction to external stimuli, such as Audit Commission reports, is purely defensive, and it is a mark of the more positive attitude in this hospital that the clinical staff saw the Commission's report as an opportunity to consider the effectiveness of the procedures in question. Indeed, Scherkenback suggests that, faced with disincentives, people tend to react predictably in what he describes as the "cycle of fear."[3] They work through three sequential phases: denial, rejecting data altogether; filtering the data, "gaming" the system by arguing

---

Organisational structure

Clinical directorate paediatrics, obstetrics and gynaecology
Chair: consultant A (paediatrician)
Members: consultant B (obstetrics and gynaecology)
community medical officer
business manager
directorate nurse
Subdirectorate obstetrics and gynaecology
Chair: consultant B
Members: consultant C
community medical officer
business manager
nurse manager
Gynaecological clinical audit group
Lead: consultant B
Support: audit assistant
All consultants and junior medical staff invited

---

about one specific data item, but ignoring the general thrust of the data; and finally, micro–management, unfocused interventions based on partial analysis of the data. These responses will be all too familiar to those working in hospitals. The case study hospital, however, had a well established culture of clinical appraisal of the services provided, based on routine analysis of appropriate, timely, and accurate information.

The debate and decision took place in the audit group which is not formally part of the management framework (box). Information focused on clinical aspects of the care regimen with an implicit acknowledgement of the resources involved. Clearly, the change in practice of the consultants would reduce pressure on beds—perhaps by the order of one or two beds over a full year. In hospitals which have devolved management responsibility to clinical management teams or directorates this freed up resource could be used to benefit the individual service, by relieving the pressure on the waiting list.

A management theorist might argue that the lack of formal linkage between the audit process and the business processes of the hospital would mean that this, and other changes in practice inspired by audit, would not be appropriately considered in

149

Audit and action

| External stimulus | Internal interest |
| (Audit Commission) | and concern |

Gather data (2 years' cases)

Analyse and review

Protocol agreed

One year

Gather data (1 year of cases)

Analyse and review

Planned further review

---

creating future year business plans and negotiating contracts. The stage at which audit information becomes management information is still a matter for debate in many hospitals.

The key to resolving this still somewhat thorny issue lies in the degree of trust and cooperation between doctors and managers in the blurring of some of the distinctions between audit and management. In compact district general hospitals overlap between the directorate and subdirectorate management groups and the audit group, through common membership, facilitates the sharing of knowledge of changes in practice. The small numbers of consultants and other staff involved also make these processes very informal. The larger hospitals, on the other hand, have experienced considerable difficulty in communicating this vital information, with its implications for the contracting process.

Whatever the size of the hospital, the clinical director must regard quality of service within the directorate as one of his or her prime responsibilities. Support from consultant colleagues with management duties in the directorate should be sought because they are in an ideal position to ensure that quality issues are progressed. Furthermore, these doctors have credibility with the medical staff to act as leads for clinical audit and can carry issues through to the management groups.

In a larger or less relaxed hospital some thought needs to be given to ensuring that the changes in clinical practice which lead to better care for individual patients are also considered in aggregate, and their overall contribution to the specialty and the

150

hospital should be considered. Information for clinical audit and information for general management are interrelated and can not be meaningfully considered in isolation.

Key point summary

- Review and analysis of retrospective patient based data can lead to changes in clinical practice, with a consequent improvement in the quality of care

- The technical ability to obtain such data and analyse them is an important component, but will not be productive without the full involvement of clinical staff

- Care needs to be taken to ensure appropriate linkages are made between clinical peer review and management mechanisms to ensure the full benefit to the organisation

- The stage at which audit information becomes management information depends on the degree of trust and cooperation between doctors and management

- "Improvement depends on learning from information about performance"[4]

---

1 Audit Commission. *A short cut to better services: day surgery in England and Wales*. London: HMSO, 1990
2 Coulter A, Klassen A, Mackenzie IZ, McPherson K. Diagnostic dilatation and curettage: is it used appropriately? *BMJ* 1993; **306**: 236-9.
3 Scherkenback WW. *The Deming route to quality and productivity*. Geo Washington University, CEE Press: 1991.
4 Berwick D. The double edge of knowledge. *J Am Med Health* 1991; **266**: 841-2.

14 The importance of quality: sharing responsibility for improving patient care

FIONA MOSS, PAM GARSIDE

In health care quality is usually understood in the context of "clinical quality" and an implicit distinction is drawn between managerial and clinical activity. The separate introduction and development of quality initiatives within the NHS has contrived to accentuate the different notions of quality that follow traditional "tribal" divisions within hospitals. Nurses often led quality assurance programmes, while doctors took up medical audit, and managers found that risk management programmes had something to offer their professional concerns. The recent directives to develop clinical audit go some way to addressing these divisions. But the onus of meeting the Patients' Charter initiatives has provided yet another separate focus for quality improvement within hospitals.

In other organisations quality improvement is often linked to the concept that quality should be a characteristic of the whole organisation. The process of quality improvement and quality control in the industrial and business world is dominated by the theory and application of total quality management (TQM). This approach to management developed after the second world war when Japanese industrialists, keen to compete with other economies, engaged American experts to advise on the application of statistical techniques to the production process. These advisors, who included W Edwards Deming and Joseph Juran, understood that documenting the technical quality or the specifications of components on a production line alone would not themselves produce lasting improvement in the quality of production. Instead, by introducing principles and techniques drawn from a wide range of disciplines, they advocated the development of an internal approach to quality improvement, where everyone in the organisation is part of a continual drive to do better. Together, these principles and techniques are described as TQM. The successful results of the application of this approach to manufacturing by the Japanese are well known.

Much has since been written on TQM and its philosophy. Some of the characteristics of TQM are shown in the box. To doctors and others working in health care much of this may be interpreted as jargon: as an approach to quality that originated in the industrial world, it has little relevance to the work of health care where customers would often rather not have the need to seek our services. The disadvantage of the divided views and approaches to quality that are endemic within the NHS is that the potential capacity of any group alone to improve quality is limited. Any approach to quality improvement in health care, to have any chance of success, has to be integrated.

The principles of TQM are far reaching and its introduction into a hospital or community trust as a mechanism for quality improvement would reqire extensive project management. It would also require long term major organisational and cultural changes, and would not be seen to satisfy the many short term pressures to improve quality that trusts are now experiencing. Nevertheless, there are lessons that can be derived from a TQM approach to quality within an organisation that are essential for developing an integrated approach to quality improvement within health care. Instituting any aspect of TQM will require trust and understanding between managers and clinical staff.

In this article we look at the necessity of management skills in the pursuit of improved quality, including the quality of clinical practice, drawing on some of the lessons from TQM. The discussion is based on a case study that incorporates three separate scenes from one hospital. We do not aim to provide all the answers, but rather to suggest approaches to improving the quality of care through a wider organisational perspective. We deliberately do not discuss all the questions raised by the case study, preferring to leave much for discussion by managers and clinicians working together in provider units.

Case study

Scene 1 – Mr Y, the outpatient services manager, has been allocated the task of meeting the Patients' Charter requirement that people should wait no longer than 30 minutes beyond their appointment time for an outpatient appointment. In one surgical clinic people waited up to two hours to see a doctor. The results of a survey done by MRY had been sent to the consultant surgeon who had written back expressing irritation and saying that if management wanted him to see more patients he needed another registrar. Meanwhile in the diabetes clinic patients were apparently being seen within 10 minutes of arrival. These figures had been collected by the diabetes care team who set and monitor their own standards, but Mr Y felt that these figures could not be correct and planned to collect his own data on that department

Scene 2 – Dr X, the clinician who leads audit in the directorate of medicine, is concerned that although three audits of the care of patients with myocardial infarction have been carried out and the results fed back to the junior staff, there has been no improvement in two important aspects of medical care. The median time between patients arriving at the hospital and receiving streptokinase remains at one hour and 20 minutes, and only 50% of patients discharged after myocardial infarction are discharged on a regimen of aspirin and a β blocker.

Scene 3 – The consultant urologists have received the length of stay data for patients admitted for transurethral prostatectomy (TURP) from the surgical business manager. They have been asked to explain the range—from five to 14 days, with a median of seven days. The urologists' first concern about these data was their accuracy. Their second was that they were already working as hard as they possibly could, as were their junior staff.

The main purchasers of care are keen to work with the hospital to improve performance in all these areas. Other possible suppliers of the surgical and urological services exist; this hospital could therefore lose some of its case load in these specialties.

The problem

These three scenes within one hospital describe the effect of dividing the responsibility for quality into sections and effectively creating systems of external inspection within an organisation in the drive for quality improvement. All the evidence from work on quality improvement suggests that this approach will not work.

The doctors in this hospital quite understandably feel threatened by receiving data that they have had no part in gathering and the implicit expectation that they have to solve "it." Mr Y is getting nowhere with waiting times in surgical outpatients and Dr X is unable to improve standards of care for patients with acute myocardial infarction. No one seems to be looking beyond their own territory to find ways of improving established deficits in care and there is an implicit assumption that the data per se will drive quality. In none of the scenes has the problem been described in terms that might suggest a solution.

Reducing waiting times in outpatient clinics, raising the standards of medical care of people with acute myocardial infarction, and minimising bed stays for people admitted with TURP are, at one level, three separate problems that need to be addressed independently by three different groups within the hospital. But there are themes common to all three: any solution will include a team approach; the needs of customers have to be understood; processes need to be changed.

The managers' role

The interest of the purchasers has forced the hospital to face up to the issues described in the case study. External pressures have also forced the hospital to look carefully at its mechanism for quality improvement. Managers within the hospital have the task of working with clinicians and others to improve performance in these individual areas. But they also need to consider the wider question of how to make the organisation less divisive. These external demands have provided the opportunity to develop some cohesion among different groups within the hospital.

Putting the patient/customer first

A fundamental principle of TQM is to put the customer first and to define quality in terms of meeting the needs of customers. In each of the scenes in the case study improvements in measurable aspects of care would clearly benefit patients/customers. The paucity of choice available to customers of health care and the dearth of information given to them about the medico-technical aspects of their care highlights

155

differences between the NHS and other organisations. The people waiting for two hours to see a surgeon in any other queue of similar length would probably have gone elsewhere. And if people with acute myocardial infarction knew about the importance of receiving thrombolytic treatment, and of the benefits of β blockers and aspirin, they would insist on receiving effective care. The new external pressures exhibited by the purchasing function and the Patients' Charter may help those working in health care to focus more on the needs of patients and other customers of health care.

TQM also recognises and emphasises the importance of internal customers within organisations. We are all, to some extent, suppliers, processors, and customers of each other's services. In this case study the surgical business manager is the supplier of information to the urologists. But the reflex doubts about the accuracy of the data suggest that in the planning of the collection of data about the length of stay of patients admitted for TURP, only scant attention was paid to involving the urologists and identifying them as "important" customers.

Understanding processes and looking at the whole picture

TQM emphasises the importance of understanding the complexity of the processes which comprise the systems for work, and emphasises that problems with quality are caused by flaws in these processes and not the people who work them. Each of these individual scenes in the case study is described one dimensionally, from the point of view of a particular service, and without an organisational perspective. Seen this way, only a limited number of options are available. The medical director and other managers need to understand each problem fully in terms of the processes or the series of steps that are needed—for example, to admit, diagnose, and treat a person admitted with acute myocardial infarction—in order to look for ways of improving the quality of care. Managers need to help the participants— consultants, junior doctors, nurses, other clinical professionals, clerks and managerial staff—to look at exactly what is being done to whom, by whom, and when.

Some of the characteristics of TQM

- Making customers' needs a priority for everyone
- Defining quality in terms of customer needs
- Recognising the existence of internal customers and suppliers
- Examining the process of production rather than individual performance for explanations of flaws or poor quality
- Using sound measurement to understand how to improve quality
- Removing barriers between staff and promoting effective team work
- Promoting training for everyone
- Involving the whole work force in the task of improving quality
- Understanding that quality improvement is a continuous process

---

Waiting times in surgical outpatients

The waiting times in the surgical outpatient clinics are unacceptable and this suggests that the clinic is poorly organised. Focusing on a single aspect of the process, such as appointment scheduling, or the work rate of the junior staff, or the time keeping of the consultant, or even the appointment of another registrar, would be unlikely to produce any major improvements. Many of the processes that are part of outpatient care can contribute to excess waiting times in clinics or waiting for first appointments. Close attention to the details of the process, some of which are a matter of clinical judgment—such as decisions about the necessity for follow up appointments—can significantly improve these aspects of outpatient practice.[1]

If the outpatient service manager could overcome his misgivings about the performance of the diabetes care team he would be able to see how another department working together as a team improved clinic waiting times. Two years ago people waited in the diabetes clinic for up to three hours and at times there were more people waiting than there were seats available. Now patients are mostly seen within 10 minutes of arrival.

Some features of diabetes care do not apply to surgical outpatient care, but much is relevant to the organisation of many outpatient services. The changes made to the organisation

157

of outpatient care for people with diabetes resulted from a detailed look at the processes of care within that department. The modifications included dividing the work into distinct groups, such as seeing new patients separately from follow up patients; giving appointment times in multiples of five minutes to suit predicted need; and incorporating the skills of nurse practitioners into the process of outpatient care.

The structure produced by these changes in the diabetes clinic allowed guidelines to be introduced to help junior doctors and has the potential to improve the training of junior staff in the outpatient care of diabetes. Of course, the structure of surgical outpatients is not the same as that of diabetes care. But once those who work in the surgical department look closely at the function and the processes of their outpatient clinic, inefficiency and wastage will be spotted and a structure that works can be developed.

Divisions between managerial and clinical activity

Doctors and other clinical professionals are the people who can make clinical decisions. Managers rely on their expertise and professional judgment. The division between managerial and clinical areas of responsibility is assumed to be clearcut. But there are interfaces where a managerial view is needed to expedite a clinical resolution. The issue of the relationship between clinical and managerial activity is not one of managers straying into professional territory, but rather a mutual understanding of the need for sound management to underpin clinical activity.

Improving the "door to needle time" for thrombolytic drugs

In this case study physicians have clearly articulated the importance of giving thrombolytic drugs to patients with myocardial infarction as soon as possible and making sure that each is discharged on a regimen of β blockers and aspirin. But, despite extensive audit, they have not managed to reduce the time it takes for patients admitted with acute myocardial infarction to receive thrombolytic drugs ("door to needle time"). Essential to the improvement of this aspect of clinical care is a close examination of the organisation of care of patients admitted with myocardial infarction. At this hospital two factors were obviously affecting the clinical management of such patients. First, it had always been hospital policy for thrombolytic drugs to be given in the coronary care unit (CCU). But the transfer time from the accident and emergency department (A and E) to CCU could take as long as 90 minutes. Secondly, all patients had to be seen by the medical registrar before thrombolytic treatment could be given. But the duty medical registrar was often in the outpatients clinic when also "on emergency take." Improvement in this aspect of the quality of clinical care will depend on substantial changes in the organisation of emergency cover. Simply feeding back audit results or issuing guidelines without attending to the organisational details will not trigger change. By changing the processes of care, one unit has reduced the "door to needle" time for thrombolytic treatment for some groups of patients from over two hours to 38 minutes.[2]

Identify team roles and professional drivers

Building effective teams is an important part of the process of quality improvement in all three scenes described in the case study. Drawing attention to the very different roles which people adopt within groups and teams, and understanding how to develop and enhance group work through recognising these differences is part of management practice.[3] Identifying the motivation of different team member and colleagues is critical as consensus cannot be built by ignoring strong individual motivations. For example, what drives urologists to manage their patients in such a way that their length of stay is twice the median? There may be justifiable reasons, but they must be examined and perhaps changed. Working properly as a team is crucial to any notion of quality improvement.

Length of stay after TURP

The urology practice of the case study illustrates an old style of approach by the clinicians. The urologists are, of course, right to challenge the accuracy of the data. But once the data are validated, to react with the "we are all working too hard" routine is inappropriate, and is not relevant to the issues presented. Looking at the problem in terms of TQM and serving the customer, the current length of stay after TURP seems arbitrary. Managers

159

have a role in facilitating the team of clinicians, including nurses and junior and senior doctors, to analyse the process of care. In the case described here all the doctors and nurses responsible for patients undergoing TURP came together to scrutinise their clinical practice. During these discussions it became apparent that minor differences in the preoperative and postoperative routine of patients undergoing TURP looked after by the two consultants were different. There was no clear set of guidelines and nurses had to wait for ward rounds for instructions to remove catheters. This delay accounted for most of the variation in length of stay. At the end of several weeks of discussion and group work the two urology firms emerged as one urology team. Conditions for removal of catheters on a fixed postoperative day had been agreed and, eventually, protocols for care of people with TURP were written and agreed. The team are now looking at the possibility of producing protocols which would serve as patient notes for both doctors and nurses.

Using this approach allowed the median length of stay for people with TURP to be reduced, and the urology team was able to produce a fact sheet for men undergoing this operation explaining the unit's routine care. This approach to reducing inpatient stays may sound straightforward, but the difficulty and pain experienced in the discussions that were needed to get this far should not be disguised nor dismissed. Encouraging and facilitating these discussions and helping with the difficulties and apparent impasses that occur is an important function, for which particular skills and aptitudes are needed.

A collective view of care, or locally developed multiprofessional guidelines, needs input from all the relevant professionals. It is not something that can be devised by managers. Such views should include those aspects of care that, based on good evidence, have important influence on outcome. Guidelines are most likely to work when developed by the team that will use them, and, some say, guidelines for medical aspects of care might function better if incorporated into multidisciplinary care plans.[4]

The importance of reliable data

Each of the scenes in the case study includes a measurement, such as length of stay, for example. One of the lessons to be derived from TQM is that good reliable data on the processes of work are necessary for quality improvement—for detecting problems; for identifying the faults in the processes; and for assessing progress. Although Dr X, in his role as clinical audit chief, had been unable to improve the timing of the administration of thrombolytic treatment, the data that had been collected were central to identifying the problem. But producing data and simply feeding them back had not promoted any change in working practice or improved quality. Moreover, it is important to make sure that data collection is one of the functions of the whole team. Presenting a surgeon with his or her outpatient waiting times without previous dicussion and agreement is unlikely to have a positive effect.

Re-evaluating the problems

The problems raised in the case study do not have a single answer that once discovered and put into action will provide a permanent solution. One of the lessons of TQM is that improving quality is a continual process which needs to become part of the routine of an organisation. This can be illustrated by looking at one of the examples in the case study, and predicting further developments.

Further improvement in "the door to needle time" for thrombolytic drugs

Changes in the medical registrar rotas, including a fixed take day and allowing thrombolytic to be given in the Accident and Emergency Department, allowed the median "door to needle" time for thrombolytic treatment to be reduced to 40 minutes. An examination of the processes of care at this stage clearly showed that most of the delays beyond one hour were occurring in cases of daignostic uncertainty and in older patients, because of a longstanding instruction that permission to give thrombolytics to older patients had to be sought from the registrar in the department of medicine for care of the elderly. Thus, as a consequence of improvements in this specific aspect of care, other problems are identified and changes to improve further the delivery of thrombolytic treatment, can be considered.

161

Conclusions

Managers in the NHS are continually forced to focus on immediate solutions to problems and have little opportunity for developing longer term organisational change. Moreover, the nature of the influence of the professions within health care produces constraints which differ from those experienced in industrial organisations. But improving quality is the concern and responsibility of all those who work in health care. This includes finding ways of working together effectively. The introduction of TQM within a health care organisation would be a daunting task, and unless this was done as part of a process which involved clinicians as well as managers it would not work. Although many of the features of TQM might seem alien to clinical practitioners, there is much within such approaches to management that would be immediately applicable to health care.[5] Quality improvement in health care is likely to be limited unless it is seen as a function of the whole organisation, and until it is realised that improvements—even in clinical quality—are most likely if managers and clinicians work together to achieve them. Managers need to explain their role and function to clinicians, and how good sound management should complement clinical practice. Clinicians need to look closely at some of their established working practices and the skills they might need to acquire to be able to work effectively in a more integrated system of health care.[6] [7]

Key point summary

- Quality improvement is on the agenda
- Total quality management has a role in the NHS
- Problems with quality are often the result of flawed processes rather than incompetent individuals
- Sound management underpins clinical activity, and the two combined effect improvements in quality
- A collective view of care requires input from all relevant professionals
- Good reliable data on the processes of work are vital
- Improving quality is a continual process

We gratefully acknowledge the helpful comments of Mr Ian Lowdon FRCS(Ed), consultant orthopaedic surgeon and medical director, Princess Margaret Hospital, Swindon.

1 NHS Executive. Outpatient attendances. *VFM Update Plus*. No 1. September 1994. London: HMSO, 1994.
2 Nee PA, Gray AJ, Martin MA. Audit of thrombolysis initiated in an accident and emergency department. *QHC* 1994; **2**: 29–33.
3 Belbin RM. Building effective management teams. *Journal of General Management* 1976; **3**: (Part 3): 23–9.
4 McNicol M, Layton A, Morgan G. Team working: the key to implementing guidelines. *QHC* 1993; **2**: 217–21.
5 Berwick DM, Godfrey AB, Roessener J. *Curing health care*. San Francisco: Jossey Bass, 1990.
6 Berwick Dm, Enthoven A, Bunker JP. Quality management in the NHS: the doctor's role—1. *BMJ* 1992; **304**: 235–9.
7 Berwick D, Enthoven A, Bunker JP. Qaulity manageent in the NHS: the doctor's role—II. *BMJ* 1992; **304**: 304–8.

15 Handling the conflicting cultures in the NHS

JAMES DRIFE, IAN JOHNSTON

Case study: working to contract

St Duncan's and St Kenneth's United Hospitals Trust, like other hospitals, is now funded by contracts which specify how much work is to be undertaken in each specialty or subspecialty. Like many hospitals in the real world outside London, the Trust has only one major purchasing authority. In the case of one specialty, ontological surgery, the volumes set for the contract are reasonable but tight.

The ontological surgeons (all men, incidentally) have always run an excellent service, including giving dates for admission within a few months to outpatients. During the year they have improved on their already impressive performance, and waiting times for admission are now a matter of weeks. The problem with this is that the hospital is now well ahead of contract and the health authority can afford to pay only for the agreed contract volumes. The health authority has also said that if it did have more money it would want to use it in specialties which were having difficulty with waiting lists.

The managerial culture requires, broadly, that the contract numbers are adhered to and the consultants have been required to restrict their activities. The doctors, however, know that there are patients waiting for treatment. They want to treat them and they believe that the health authority's problems are not theirs. They feel that if other specialties have excessive waiting lists they should be required to get their house in order before being given extra funds. The managers and the doctors have reached an impasse.

The NHS is a multicultural society. Each profession—medical, nursing, management and many others—has its own identity, culture, and subcultures. Within medicine there are various specialty groupings, such as surgeons, psychiatrists, or GPs, with different characteristics and aims. The potential for conflict arising from cultural differences is almost limitless—a problem not, of course, unique to the NHS.[1] This chapter focuses as an example on the relationship between NHS managers and doctors and concentrates on conflict and its resolution. The overall relationship is a much richer subject than can be addressed here and it has been well discussed by Harrison[2] as well as by other authors in this series.

The tension between the amount of clinical work that could be done and the amount of money available to pay for it has always been present in the NHS. The recent reforms have highlighted the differences between medical and management responses to this tension.

To handle this conflict successfully, each group needs to understand the other's culture. Often they think they do, but what understanding they have may be based on stereotype and often tends to reinforce rather than reduce antagonism.

The managers' view

From the manager's perspective this matter may seem eminently clear. The contract volumes have been agreed and therefore have to be maintained. Despite much opinion to the contrary, managerial life is not as simple as that. Managers are public servants and take their responsibilities to the public seriously. They know that someone has to take on the task of ensuring that all the demands of politicians, doctors, patients, therapists, nurses, etc, are balanced and health care is delivered as equitably as possible.

The hospital managers know that life is more complicated than the ontological surgeons allow. The managers, like the surgeons, are on the patients' side but they also know that choices have to be made and priorities agreed. Unfettered developments in ontology will lead to problems for the patients of other specialties—apparently beyond the immediate concerns of the ontological surgeons.

The managerial perspective does indeed accept that contracts have to be kept. What kind of world would it be if they were routinely flouted? How could any hospital survive and flourish if its key staff ignored what had been agreed? From this point of view the failure lies squarely with the consultants for not planning their work for the year. It cannot be denied that not only is such planning possible but these consultants are good at it.

Any manager must recognise what has been achieved by the consultants. From the patients' and the general practitioners' point of view this specialty is a success. The managerial perspective also requires that the service's users remain satisfied. It will be of no benefit to the hospital if such a highly successful service is seen as being curtailed or cut. The manager understands that except for the use of draconian measures it is only through the cooperation of the consultants that any change to this service can occur. (For an analysis of control mechanisms and clinical freedom, see Harrison.[3])

Yet action must be taken. The hospital cannot do work for which it is not paid. To allow the present position to continue in this specialty would lead to financial difficulties. If no action is taken here other specialties will follow suit and the whole hospital will face financial crisis.

The doctors' view

The ontological surgeons know that working to contract means treating fewer patients than they want to treat, and therefore either working less during the normal week or stopping completely as the end of the financial year approaches. They find this unacceptable because of their traditional work ethic and because they want to help people. In the main GPs address referral letters not to the manager but personally to the consultant. A deterioration in the hospital service harms the surgeon's reputation, which has taken years to build up.

More altruistically, he feels angry on the patient's behalf. He has found that prompt service usually surprises his patients, who expect to queue for NHS treatment and rarely complain if they are forced to wait. The consultants feel that they alone are responsible for maintaining good standards. This leads to the "mother tiger" syndrome, with a ferocious doctor trying to protect the interests of docile patients.

The ontologists are not convinced that the hospital will suffer if they continue to work. The biggest cost in a hospital is the staff. Surgeons, anaesthetists, and nurses are not being made redundant; the beds are there and the ward is being heated and lit. Why, then, will an operation that uses relatively little consumable material cost the accountant so much money? The surgeons feel the accountant's perception has little to do with real life.

Doctors feel aloof from imperatives that affect managers. Regarding themselves as being at the apex of the hospital hierarchy, they are not overawed by top management. They see contracts and purchaser/provider arrangements as an irrelevance. Even if the entire NHS collapses, their clinical work will continue because a new system will be created around them.

The ontological surgeons feel they have the support of colleagues in other professions. The operating theatre, despite being a mixture of cultures, works like a military unit. The bonding in a surgical team can be as strong as that in a platoon in battle—while it is under attack from a common enemy. Relationships between the cultures may be complex in the team but the team unites against perceived threats from outside.

Handling the conflict

There are many ways in which conflict between cultures can be handled.[1 4] At one extreme is the use of power to assert the rightness of one approach over the other. This is generally tactfully deployed, but this method of resolving conflicts is nevertheless quite common. However, in a complex and changing environment like the NHS, where allies will always be needed in future conflicts, it is more common to see such approaches reduced to compromise. The "deals" which conflicting parties reach are a tacit recognition that no profession or culture is totally dominant. Resolution of conflict in this way is always incomplete: more deals will be needed before too long.

It is a fact of life that most conflict is "handled" and little is resolved. Differences create progress and organisations which manage conflict constructively are the ones that make the greatest progress.[5] We are optimistic about the possibilities. Most conflicts as they occur day to day in the NHS could be resolved if the will and understanding were really there. The fact that they are not reflects a general belief that it is not possible and that the cultures in the NHS are irresolvably in conflict. In particular, the belief is becoming entrenched that conflict between managers and doctors is somehow an intrinsic part of the NHS. We believe this is neither desirable nor necessary. What are the steps out of eternal conflict?

Step 1: mutual respect

The first essential is mutual respect between the parties. That is, an acceptance of the legitimacy of the separate cultures and an acceptance that other people really do hold to their beliefs as strongly as you. To achieve this needs time, effort, and communication skills. You can accept another culture only if you understand it, and you cannot understand it if you stay locked within your own culture and simply reinforce your own prejudices. Doctors and nurses talk to each other every day; even so, cultural misunderstanding persists. It is rare for doctors and managers to enjoy lunch or a tea break together, except at formal meetings. It is essential to allow sufficient time for this informal interaction.

Step 2: shared values

Following mutual acceptance, it is possible to define the values which both cultures share.[6] This requires tenacity, as discussions between managers and doctors tend to gravitate towards areas of disagreement. All too often each party seizes on inconsistencies in the other's statements, and discussion sometimes resembles the presentations of opposing counsel in court—but with no judge to arbitrate. Keeping the discussion focused on shared values means stating these values explicitly and honestly, and restating them as often as necessary.

In the present case what can be shared is a desire to provide good care, and for the hospital to thrive as a whole. Political beliefs can be acknowledged but must not be allowed to polarise local discussions. Neither doctors nor managers want to turn the ontology service into a political football. Both recognise that they have to work within a democracy, and that the democratic process legitimately leads to changing requirements from its health care system.

Step 3: honesty

Discussions between managers and doctors have for years been characterised by poker playing. Each side takes up a negotiating position but has a fallback position which is what it usually expects. This can lead doctors into shroud waving and over-bidding for equipment, and cause managers to overstate the size of the hospital's overdraft. Sooner or later the bluff is revealed and from then on neither group believes a word the other says. The problem with lying as routine has been well illustrated by Aesop in his fable about the boy who cried wolf. We suggest that it is time to learn this 2500 year old lesson. Honesty is the best policy, even when doctors and managers meet.

Step 4: shared objectives

Based on values which both cultures share it is then possible to agree shared objectives about the way forward. (For a framework of values and its relationship to organisation development, see Kinston.[7]) The first step is to discuss all possible hidden objectives. One way of stimulating frank discussion is to breach etiquette by putting the hidden agenda on the table. Do the managers want to make a point about who is in charge of the hospital? Do the surgeons want to provoke a public confrontation so as to involve the electorate at large in the debate about NHS funding? If these threatening options are made explicit they can be examined objectively. After discussion they are likely to be rejected.

The doctors and managers can then agree short term and medium term objectives. In the case study the short term objective will be agreement on the immediate workload and the medium term objective is to decide the level of next year's contract. In the long term, who knows?—perhaps sharing values and agreeing objectives will provide the foundations to deal with whatever changes occur to the NHS in the future.

Step 5: combating disinformation

Once initial agreement is reached by representative groups, they must convince their sceptical colleagues—that is to say, the values and objectives must be truly shared. Hospital gossip tends to reduce issues to simplistic conflict and unfortunately, in many places conflict has more credibility than consensus. Managers' cheerful newsheets are often perceived as propaganda and have to be backed up by word of mouth. A modern hospital, like eighteenth century London, is a coffee house culture and mutual respect and shared values cannot survive for long if they are undermined by off the record chat. Both doctors and managers, having emerged with consensus from a constructive discussion, may be tempted to impress their respective peers by claiming a victory against the old enemy, thus reducing the danger of their being seen as traitors to their own culture. A little of this may be necessary to avoid cultural isolation, but more than a little is counterproductive and undermines any progress made.

Conclusion

Our steps may seem to be compromise with a different hat on. They are, however, conceptually very different. Compromise is based on the balance of power and is therefore unstable because power relations change. The approach we are advocating is based on values and values endure. It applies not only to doctors and managers but to other cultures within the NHS, all of which—despite their conflicts—share similar enduring values.

Key point summary

- Mutual respect is essential between management and clinicians and other health care professionals

- Shared values need to be expressed explicitly and honestly, and frequently restated

- Shared objectives need to be identified

- Disinformation should be combated

---

1 Handy CB. On politics and the management of differences. In: *Understanding organisations* 3rd edn. Harmondsworth: Penguin, 1998: 222–56.
2 Harrison S. *Managing the NHS: shifting the frontier?* London: Chapman & Hall, 1988.
3 Harrison S. The frontier of control. In: *Managing the NHS: shifting the frontier?* London: Chapman & Hall, 1988: 1–8.
4 Mintzberg H. *Power in and around organisations.* New York: Prentice–Hall, 1983.
5 Lickert R. The principles of supportive relationships. In: Pugh DS, ed. *Organisation theory—selected readings.* Harmondsworth: Penguin, 1987: 293–316.
6 Kinston W. *Strengthening the management culture.* London. The Sigma Centre, 1994.
7 Kinston W. The rationalist mode. In: *Strengthening the management culture.* London: The Sigma Centre, 1994: 43–53.

Index